To my husband Will, for his endless patience and for enabling me to fulfil my dreams. I must also thank my children, Daniel, Steven, Natasha and Belinda who have never once complained about the hours Mummy has spent working. Finally, to Jim for giving me the opportunity.

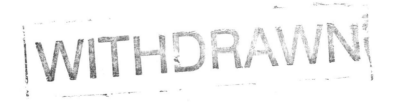

Contents

Preface

This book is written with the intention of providing nurse practitioners working in the field of acute medicine with an up-to-date, practical and comprehensive guide to the management of acute medical patients.

It is hoped that it will serve as a text from which the busy, highly skilled nurse can obtain information on the assessment, investigation, diagnosis and management of acute medical conditions.

In my role as Consultant Nurse in Acute Medicine I appreciate the diversity this speciality brings and the challenges faced by working at an advanced level in this acute environment.

This book aims to provide the reader with an evidence-based approach to the management of the most common medical conditions.

Introduction

No man not even a Doctor expects a nurse to be anything other than this – devoted and obedient.

Florence Nightingale, 1887

Nursing has changed dramatically since the days of Florence Nightingale. Traditional doctor/nurse boundaries are being eroded and nurses are expanding their sphere of practice to encompass assessment skills and to enable them to manage total episodes of patient care with true autonomy (DOH 2000). More recently we have seen the emergence of nurse practitioners undertaking this advanced level of health assessment in the acute medical arena. This book is intended to support the decision-making process and treatment that can be offered by these individuals.

The book takes the reader through the assessment, investigation, diagnosis and management of the most common acute medical conditions. It identifies priorities for treatment and guides the reader through the management of the patient. Wherever possible the latest published guidelines have been included.

The final chapter of the book considers the legal, professional and ethical issues faced by nurses working at an advanced level. The issues of role development, the development of protocols and prescribing are considered.

At the back of the book are examples of Clinical Management Plans for the supplementary prescriber and Patient Group Directions to support practice. There is also a glossary to explain terms and to serve as a useful reference guide.

This book will provide invaluable information and advice to the established and aspiring practitioner working in the field of acute medicine.

1 Patient Assessment

The general public have an expectation that when they are unwell they will be assessed by a competent practitioner who will be able to tell them what is wrong and treat the problem. As a nurse practitioner working in an acute medical environment such as a medical assessment unit this expectation becomes your remit.

In order to provide a patient with a diagnosis and treatment it is necessary to undertake a detailed history and physical assessment. Therefore the importance of the history cannot be overestimated. Patients need to feel at ease and able to discuss their health concerns and problems with the practitioner, and therefore a good 'bedside manner' is vital. With this in mind this chapter will discuss communication skills and general hints on preparing a patient for assessment. The medical model of history-taking and assessment, along with the more nursing-orientated SOAPIE model of assessment, will be discussed. Towards the end of this chapter, hints can be found on a systems approach to physical assessment.

COMMUNICATION

Good communication with a patient enables a relationship of trust to develop. Patients need to know that they can trust the practitioner delivering their care. Good communication improves health outcomes. This can lead to the resolution of symptoms, fewer adverse psychological effects and a reduction in pain levels. Poor communication leads to a patient feeling devalued and vulnerable (Longmore et al. 2001). Most complaints in healthcare do not arise as a result of poor clinical care or omission but as a result of poor communication. In other words, the patient did not know what was happening to them. Perhaps a good motto to remember is: 'How would I feel if this was me or a relative of mine?' If you were not satisfied with the answers or explanations that you have just given, why should the patient be? Following some straightforward general rules during any consultation with patients will help improve communication.

- *Always introduce yourself.* Patients like to know who is asking them questions and examining them. Remember to introduce yourself as a nurse, especially if you don't wear uniform. The public still make an assumption that anyone wearing normal clothes and carrying a stethoscope must be a doctor. Medico-legally it is important that they know you are a nurse. Experience will tell you that the patient may still call you 'doctor' despite your efforts to explain differently. Take it as a compliment!

- *Make sure your patient is comfortable.* An uncomfortable patient is not going to answer questions in any detail. Help them into a position that is most comfortable for them.
- *Ensure privacy.* This is often difficult in an acute environment such as a medical assessment unit. Always close the curtains and remember that they are not a barrier to what is being said. Other patients will be able to hear both the questions asked and the answers given. There is no easy solution to this. The demands of an acute environment are such that it is not always possible to move a patient into an area where they are alone with you. Be sensitive to this. If you need to ask extremely personal questions – for example, questioning about sexual activity and sexual partners – it may be pertinent to arrange to move the patient to a more private area, or make a decision as to whether or not you need the answer to that particular question immediately or if it can wait until a later stage. Privacy can be difficult in situations where your patient is extremely deaf, resulting in the need to raise your voice, almost to shouting on occasions. This does not ensure confidentiality or privacy for the patient. Discuss with management the purchase of patient handheld amplifiers which can resolve this problem.
- *Ensure dignity is maintained and be culturally aware.* Always maintain your patient's dignity. During physical examination the patient does not need to be naked and fully exposed. Expose the parts you wish to examine in turn. Remember, what would you want if it was you or your relative? Ask the question, do you need a chaperone? This is not just relevant for men examining women but equally as important to consider when you are a woman examining a man. Considerations should include the age of the patient, the vulnerability of the patient (old, young, learning disabilities, mental health problems) and the patient's wishes. Be culturally aware. It may, for example, be unacceptable for a young woman from certain cultures to be examined by a man. Ask the patient if it is alright for you to examine them. If they wish to be examined by someone of the same sex as themselves you must ensure that this happens.
- *Explain to the patient what is going to happen.* This may sound obvious but it is an important part of putting the patient at ease. Start by explaining that you are going to ask them some questions about what has been happening recently and led up to their admission, and that you will then need to know about their past medical history. Explain that you will then examine them and after this they will have some tests which will help decide on treatment. Let the patient know that you will keep them informed of what is happening throughout this process. Make sure you tell the patient that while all this is happening you will be making notes. Unless it is an emergency situation, always write things down as you go along. Leaving it until the end inevitably results in having to return to the patient to ask a question again as you have forgotten what they said the first time. This is frustrating for all involved and does not inspire confidence.
- *Avoid jargon.* As practitioners we are used to medical terminology but it is a foreign language for most patients. Keep it simple. This may sound like common sense but we have all witnessed the scenario where the consultant sees a patient on the ward

round, leaves the bedside and the patient then asks the nurse what the consultant has just said. Using simple terminology is more likely to result in getting the answers to your questions. If a patient answers a question using medical jargon, clarify what they mean. Patients often use medical terms incorrectly. Be specific and never assume that your patient can read.

- *Listen to your patient.* If you ask the right questions in the right way you will get the answers. The days of the patient doing exactly what they were told by the team looking after them simply because they must know best are long gone. In this day and age we aim for concordance not compliance. *Compliance* implies a medical-led approach to care. The practitioner says 'Take this' and the patient does so. *Concordance* means developing a partnership with patients. The patient has the options explained and has some understanding of treatments and how they work and why they need to take them. The healthcare professional and the patient devise a treatment plan that suits the patient and treats the problem appropriately. If you do not listen to your patient you will not achieve concordance.

HISTORY TAKING

THE SOAPIE MODEL

As a nurse practitioner it is vital that you can take a history in a structured format. Many nurses in expanded roles have adopted the traditional medical model of history taking. The medical model is an established, structured approach that all health care disciplines are used to reading. It may be that you are already using or may decide to follow the medical model, and this is perfectly acceptable. It is important that any decision made is an informed one, hence the inclusion of the SOAPIE model in this section.

As nurses we are used to the assess, plan, implement, evaluate approach to health care. The SOAPIE model maintains this approach while incorporating elements of the medical model (Welsby 2002). SOAPIE stands for:

Subjective data
Objective data
Assessment
Plan
Implementation
Evaluation

- *Subjective data* – obtaining information on the presenting problem. The focus of this enquiry is to ascertain what the patient states the problem is. What are their symptoms?
- *Objective data* – what you the practitioner find as a result of observation, direct questioning and physical examination. The line of direct questioning may follow that of a medical model.

- *Assessment* – your physical assessment. This may follow a medical model structure.
- *Plan* – your proposed plan of care. This will include both the medical and nursing plan of care.
- *Implementation* – what you have done for the patient and what you require others to do.
- *Evaluation* – how effective has the treatment/care been? At this stage it may be necessary to return to the objective data and assessment and revise the plan.

THE MEDICAL MODEL

The medical model is, as already stated, a tried and tested method of assessment and in many ways is very similar to the SOAPIE model as subjective and objective data are collated, the physical assessment follows and a treatment plan is devised (Bates 1995; Longmore et al. 2001). As a nurse practitioner whichever model you decide to utilise it is important that you ensure assessment and plans of care cover both the nursing and medical aspects.

The medical model follows a very logical approach:

Presenting complaint – what has brought the patient to seek help.

- What do they say is wrong with them?
- What are the patient's symptoms?

History of presenting complaint – use direct questioning to find out:

- When the problem started.
- How it has progressed.
- If they have ever had anything like it before.

Whichever model you decide to use, if the patient has pain it may be useful to use the acronym SOCRATES to aid assessment.

Site – if possible get the patient to show you where it hurts.
Onset – when did it start? Was it gradual or sudden?
Character – is the pain sharp, stabbing, a heaviness?
Radiation – does the pain go anywhere else?
Associated features – e.g. shortness of breath, nausea, vomiting, sweating.
Timing – when did it come on? How long have they had it for?
Exacerbating/relieving factors – what makes it worse/better, have they taken anything?
Severity – on a scale of 1–10 (10 being the worst).

Past medical history – do they have any other illnesses?

- List illnesses in a language the patient can understand such as diabetes, heart attack, asthma, emphysema, epilepsy, high blood pressure, angina, jaundice, anaemia, tuberculosis.
- Ask if they have ever been in hospital before.
- Have they had any operations?

Medications and allergies – ask if they take any medications.

- Don't forget to ask about over the counter drugs and complementary therapies.
- Make a list of the medications, dosage and frequency if the patient has the tablets with them or a list from their GP. If this is not available, make it your responsibility to contact the GP when you have finished seeing the patient or ensure it is handed over for someone to obtain this information at the earliest opportunity.
- Ask about allergies. If the patient states they have an allergy to a drug or substance, ask them what happens when they take the drug or come into contact with the substance. Many people state they have an allergy when in fact it was a side effect of the treatment.

Severe allergic reactions can be classified in three stages of severity:

A – an allergy causing an airway problem
B – an allergy causing a breathing problem
C – an allergy causing a circulatory problem

Allergic reactions that cause symptoms such as rash, running nose, diarrhoea and vomiting are classified as mild reactions.

Ascertain whether the patient has ever been tested by a doctor for allergies and whether they carry an EpiPen. If they carry an EpiPen have they ever had to use it?

Social and family history

- Who do they live with?
- Do they have help with shopping, cleaning etc?
- Is a care package in place?
- Have there been any recent trips abroad? If so, where did they go and did they receive any vaccinations?
- At this stage it is important to know if they smoke. If so, how many do they smoke a day and for how many years have they smoked? Work out the pack years (NICE 2004):

$$\text{Total pack years} = \frac{\text{number smoked per day}}{20} \times \text{number of years smoked}$$

- It is important to ascertain what the patient does or did for a living. Certain jobs may increase an individual's risk of certain diseases. For example, a pottery worker or miner may have industrial lung disease.
- If they have been a miner, do they get a pension and if so what percentage? The higher percentage pension they receive the more severe their lung disease as a result of working in the mines. Other industries that may have an occupational health hazard associated with them include: the armed forces, agriculture, stone masons and arc welders.
- Ask if they have ever knowingly been exposed to asbestos.
- When taking a social history, do not forget to ask about alcohol consumption, both past and present.

- Ask about pets at home, particularly bird-keeping which can precipitate lung disease.
- It is important to ascertain if there is a history of drug abuse and in some circumstances obtain a sexual history. However, be sensitive and use your clinical judgement to decide whether or not you believe these questions are pertinent at this particular time.

Once this has been ascertained it is important to recap on anything which you remain unclear about. It is then time to move on to the functional enquiry and the physical assessment.

THE FUNCTIONAL ENQUIRY

The functional enquiry is the time when you ask questions about each of the body systems before you begin the physical examination. Start with some general questions before going on to each system in turn (Bates 1995; Longmore et al. 2001; Welsby 2002).

GENERAL QUESTIONS

- Ask the patient if they are concerned about anything in particular.
- Have they lost weight recently? If the answer is yes it is important to ascertain if this has been intentional. If the answer is no proceed to ask if they have gained weight; if so, how much, over what period of time?
- Ascertain what their appetite is like. If they have lost their appetite, do they not feel hungry, does food cause them to feel sick, be sick, or give them pain?
- Have they noticed any unusual lumps anywhere in their body recently? If so, where are they and when did they first notice them? You can examine them later.
- Have they noticed any night sweats? If yes, when did they start, how regularly do they occur, do they have to change their night clothes and bed sheets?
- Have they noticed any unusual rashes? Have they felt particularly itchy recently?

CARDIORESPIRATORY SYMPTOMS

- If you have not already asked about chest pain, now is the time to do so. Remember SOCRATES.
- Have they experienced any palpitations? If yes, are they regular or irregular? If possible get the patient to tap them out to you.
- Ask about shortness of breath. If they get short of breath, how far can they walk now before getting short of breath? It is quite useful to give them examples such as 'Could you walk from here to the door?' It may be helpful to ask the patient to cast their mind back six months. What was their breathing like six months ago? How far could they walk then? What is their breathing like going up stairs / up hills? Do they need to stop?

- Do they wake up in the night short of breath (paroxysmal nocturnal dyspnoea)? Does it feel as if they can't get air into the lungs? Do they need to get to the window and open it?
- How many pillows do they sleep with? Has this number increased? Do they get short of breath if they lie flat (orthopnoea)?
- Have they noticed any swelling of their legs? Is it both legs or only one leg that swells? Is this something new or an ongoing problem?
- Have they got a cough? Are they expectorating any sputum? If yes, what colour is it? Is it associated with a foul taste or smell? How long have they had it? Have they been given any treatment by their GP?
- Have they noticed a wheeze when breathing? If yes, when did it start? Is it worse at any particular time of day? Is it made worse by exercise?

GASTROINTESTINAL SYMPTOMS

You will have already asked some general questions about weight loss and appetite in general questions. Now is the time to get more detail.

- Ask about abdominal pain. If the patient has abdominal pain you can use the SOCRATES model to assess the pain in detail. When utilising this model remember abdominal pain can be described as colicky, sharp, stabbing and dull. When asking about associated features discuss in particular nausea, vomiting and bowel movements. The same applies to exacerbating and relieving factors.
- Ask about indigestion, nausea and vomiting. If the patient complains of indigestion is this worse before or after eating and does anything help to relieve the discomfort?
- Is there any difficulty in swallowing? Does it feel as if food gets stuck? If so, ask the patient to show you where the food seems to get stuck. Is the problem with liquids and solids or with just one of these?
- Ask if there are any problems with bowel movements. If the patient states they have diarrhoea or constipation, clarify what they mean by this. Many patients will state they have diarrhoea when in fact this is not the case. Remember, diarrhoea is defined as the passage of frequent watery stools. It is also important to ascertain if there has been any altered bowel habit.
- It is important to ascertain what the stool is like. What is the colour and consistency? Does the stool contain any blood? If yes, is it fresh blood, or is the stool black? Ask yourself, is the patient taking any iron preparations? Does the patient complain of tenesmus – a feeling that there is something in the rectum which cannot be passed?

GENITO-URINARY SYMPTOMS

You may already have been given some hint as to whether or not your patient has any GU symptoms from previous questions. Below are some thoughts to guide your questioning further.

- Does the patient have any GU symptoms? Are they suffering from incontinence? If they are incontinent, is this stress or urge incontinence?
- Stress incontinence is due to an incompetent sphincter. Urge incontinence occurs when the urge to pass urine is quickly followed by the uncontrollable complete emptying of the bladder as the detrousor muscle contracts. The main cause of incontinence in men is enlargement of the prostate gland causing urge incontinence.

NEUROLOGICAL SYMPTOMS

As with all the other systems enquiries, you may already have some answers to these questions.

- Ask about the five senses – sight, hearing, taste, smell and touch.
- Has vision deteriorated? If yes, over what period of time? Is there any double vision? Any blurred vision?
- Is hearing affected? Has there been a loss of hearing? If yes, is it in both ears or one? Any tinitus?
- Have taste and smell altered? Again, you want to know when this started and how it has altered. Have they noticed any altered sensation in any part of their body? Any limb weakness, loss of power?
- Ask about headache – if the patient has a headache use SOCRATES to guide your questioning.
- Ask about speech difficulties – dysphasia and dysarthria.
  - ➢ *Dysphasia* – impairment of language caused by damage to the brain. The patient will have difficulty in producing fluent speech, words may be malformed. The patient does not have any difficulty comprehending what is being said to them, but reading and writing are impaired and this frequently leads to frustration. Dysphasia manifests itself in varying degrees of severity from those with very mild symptoms to those that are very severe.
  - ➢ *Dysarthria* – this is difficulty with articulation and is due to a lack of co-ordination or weakness of the muscle used in speech. Language is perfectly normal. This may manifest itself as slurring of speech, slow or indistinct speech.
- Ask about seizures – frequency, diurnal variation, anything that provokes a seizure? A witness account of seizure activity is always helpful.

MUSCULOSKELETAL SYMPTOMS

- Are joints painful? You can use SOCRATES.
- Is there any stiffness or swelling of joints?
- Is there any diurnal variation in symptoms?
- How does all this affect activities of daily living?

THE PHYSICAL ASSESSMENT

It is important to continue to utilise a structured approach to the physical assessment. Once you have found a system that works for you, stick to it. This ensures that you will not miss anything (Longmore et al. 2001).

This is an ideal opportunity to clarify anything that you are still not clear about following the functional enquiry. You can continue to talk to the patient about their symptoms while you are examining them.

Physical assessment utilises four basic techniques:

1. inspection
2. palpation
3. percussion
4. auscultation

- Always assess in this order except when examining the abdomen.
- Use each technique to compare symmetrical sides of the body and organs.
- Assess both structure and function.

1. INSPECTION

This is the observation of various body parts using the senses of sight, hearing and smell to detect normal functioning or any deviations from normal.

Technique

- Exposure of appropriate body part.
- Always look before you touch.
- Use good lighting.
- Ensure warm environment.
- Observe for colour, size, location, texture, symmetry, odours and sounds.

2. PALPATION

This is the touching and feeling of various body parts with the hands to determine certain characteristics:

- texture
- temperature
- moisture
- movement
- consistency of structures

Technique

- Short fingernails are important.
- Use appropriate part of hand to detect different sensations:

> fingertips – fine discriminations / pulsations.
> palmar surface – vibratory sensations.
> dorsal surface – temperature.
- Palpate lightly first then deeply.
- Any tender areas should be left until last.
- There are three types of palpation:
  > light palpation.
  > deep palpation.
  > bimanual palpation.

3. PERCUSSION

This is to tap a portion of the body to detect any tenderness or sounds which will vary with the density of underlying structures.

Technique

Direct:

- Tap an area with 1–2 fingertips.

Indirect:

- Place middle finger of non-dominant hand on body.
- Keep other fingers out of the way.
- Tap middle finger with middle finger of dominant hand quickly.
- Listen to sound.

4. AUSCULTATION

The use of a stethoscope to detect various breath, heart and bowel sounds.

Technique

Use a good stethoscope with:

- snug-fitting ear pieces
- tubing no longer than 15 ins (38 cm) with an internal diameter not greater than $1/8$ in (0.3 cm)
- bell and diaphragm

Diaphragm and bell are used for detecting different sounds:

- diaphragm – for high-pitched sounds, i.e. breath sounds, normal heart and bowel sounds
- bell – for low-pitched sounds, i.e. abnormal heart sounds and bruits

Percussion note	Origin	Sound	Example
Tympany	Enclosed air	Drum like	Gas in bowel Puffed out cheek
Resonance	Part air/part solid	Hollow	Normal lung
Hyper-resonance	Increased air in solid tissue	Booming	Lung with emphysema
Dullness	More solid tissue	Thud sound	Internal organs (not lung)
Flatness	Very dense tissue	Flat	Bone, muscle

Figure 1.1. Percussion note table.

GENERAL INSPECTION

DEMEANOUR

- Observe gait.
- Facial expressions.
- Facial responses to your questions.

PHYSIQUE

- Assess build.
- Is their physique balanced.
- Does physique of upper body match that of the lower body.

GENERAL CONDITION

- Note nutritional state.
- Height, weight and BMI (if possible).
- Hydration – skin turgor, orbital pressure (not in glaucoma) and mucous membranes.
- Speech.
- Abnormal sounds – hoarseness of voice.
- Borborygmi (growling bowel sounds).
- Abnormal odours.

GENERAL SIGNS

- Inspect for signs of peripheral and central cyanosis.
- Look for signs of clubbing – an exaggerated longitudinal curvature and loss of the angle between the nail and nail fold. The nail feels 'boggy'.
- Check capillary refill time. A normal capillary refill time is <2 seconds.
- Inspect for signs of peripheral oedema.
- Check radial pulses bilaterally.

- Record blood pressure.
- Record oxygen saturations.
- Record peak expiratory flow.

RESPIRATORY EXAMINATION

INSPECTION

- Observe the rate, rhythm, depth and effort of breathing.
- Listen for abnormal sounds with breathing such as wheezes.
- Observe for use of accessory muscles.
- Look for signs of asymmetry and deformity.
- Is the trachea central?
- Is there any evidence of tracheal decent?

PALPATION

- Identify any areas of tenderness or deformity by palpating the ribs and sternum.
- Assess expansion and symmetry of the chest by placing your hands on the patient's back, thumbs together at the midline, and asking them to breathe deeply.
- Check for tactile fremitus.
- Palpate for cervical lymphadenopathy.

PERCUSSION

Posterior Chest

- Percuss from side to side and top to bottom.
- Compare one side to the other looking for asymmetry.
- Note the location and quality of the percussion sounds you hear.
- Find the level of the diaphragmatic dullness on both sides.

Diaphragmatic Excursion

- Find the level of the diaphragmatic dullness on both sides.
- Ask the patient to inspire deeply.
- The level of dullness (diaphragmatic excursion) should go down by 3–5 cm symmetrically.

Anterior Chest

- Percuss from side to side and top to bottom. Compare one side to the other, looking for asymmetry.
- Note the location and quality of the percussion sounds you hear.

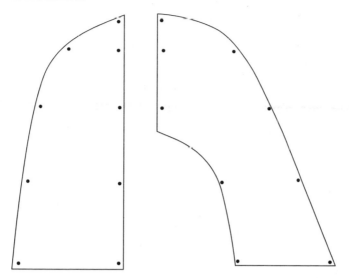

Figure 1.2. Posterior chest examination.

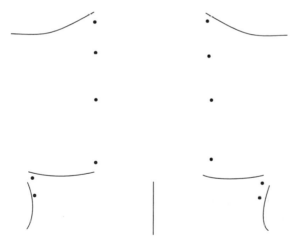

Figure 1.3. Anterior chest examination.

Percussion notes and their meaning	
Flat or dull	Pleural effusion or lobar pneumonia
Normal	Healthy lung or bronchitis
Hyperresonant	Emphysema or pneumothorax

Figure 1.4. Percussion note interpretation table.

Abnormal lung sounds	
Crackles	These are high-pitched, discontinuous sounds similar to the sound produced by rubbing your hair between your fingers (also known as Rales)
Wheezes	These are generally high pitched and 'musical' in quality. Stridor is an inspiratory wheeze associated with upper airway obstruction (croup)
Rhonchi	These often have a 'snoring' or 'gurgling' quality. Any extra sound that is not a crackle or a wheeze is probably a rhonchi

Figure 1.5. Interpretation of abnormal lung sounds.

AUSCULTATION

Posterior Chest

• Auscultate from side to side and top to bottom (see Figures 1.2 and 1.3).
• Compare one side to the other, looking for asymmetry.
• Note the location and quality of the sounds you hear.

Anterior Chest

• Auscultate from side to side and top to bottom (see Figures 1.2 and 1.3).
• Compare one side to the other, looking for asymmetry.
• Note the location and quality of the sounds you hear.

CARDIOVASCULAR EXAMINATION

GENERAL INSPECTION

If not already done:

• assess for signs of peripheral and central cyanosis
• observe for signs of clubbing
• check capillary refill time
• record blood pressure
• record pulse (see Figure 1.6)

Rate and Rhythm of Arterial Pulses

• Compress the radial artery with your index and middle fingers.
• Note whether the pulse is regular or irregular.

Normal pulse rate	60–100 beats per minute
Bradycardia	Less than 60 beats per minute
Tachycardia	Greater than 100 beats per minute

Figure 1.6. Heart rate table.

Regular rhythm	Evenly spaced beats – may vary slightly with inspiration
Regularly irregular	Regular pattern with regular skipped or extra beats
Irregularly irregular	No pattern. Atrial fibrillation – always record apex beat for 1 minute

Figure 1.7. Heart rhythm table.

- Count for a full minute if the pulse is irregular and record apex rate.
- Record the rate and rhythm.

Auscultation for Bruits

- Auscultate for bruits.
- Place the bell of the stethoscope over each carotid artery in turn.
- Ask the patient to stop breathing momentarily.
- Listen for a blowing or rushing sound – a bruit.

Jugular Venous Pressure

- Position the patient supine with the head of the table elevated 45°.
- Look for a rapid, double (sometimes triple) wave with each heart beat.
- Identify the highest point of pulsation.
- Using a horizontal line from this point, measure vertically from the sternal angle.
- This measurement should be less than 4 cm in a normal healthy adult.

AUSCULTATION

- Position the patient supine with the head of the table slightly elevated (see Figure 1.8).
- Listen with the diaphragm at the right 2nd intercostal space near the sternum (aortic area).
- Listen with the diaphragm at the left 2nd intercostal space near the sternum (pulmonary area).
- Listen with the diaphragm at the left 3rd, 4th, and 5th intercostal spaces near the sternum (tricuspid area).
- Listen with the diaphragm at the apex (mitral area). Apex beat should be heard at the 5th intercostal space in the mid clavicluar line.
- Listen with the bell at the apex.
- Listen with the bell at the left 4th and 5th intercostal space near the sternum.
- Ask the patient to roll onto their left side.
- Listen with the bell at the apex. This position brings out S3 and mitral murmurs.

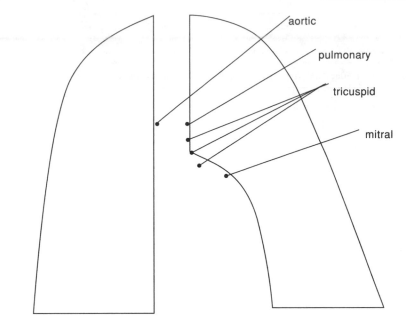

aortic

pulmonary

tricuspid

mitral

Figure 1.8. Cardiovascular examination.

- Ask the patient to sit up, lean forward, and hold their breath in exhalation.
- Listen with the diaphragm at the left 3rd and 4th intercostal space near the sternum. This position brings out aortic murmurs.
- Record all heart sounds including any murmurs heard and the severity of the murmur.

Murmur grades		
Grade	**Volume**	**Thrill**
1/6	very faint, only heard with optimal conditions	no
2/6	loud enough to be obvious	no
3/6	louder than grade 2	no
4/6	louder than grade 3	yes
5/6	heard with the stethoscope partially off the chest	yes
6/6	heard with the stethoscope completely off the chest	yes

Figure 1.9. Heart murmurs table.

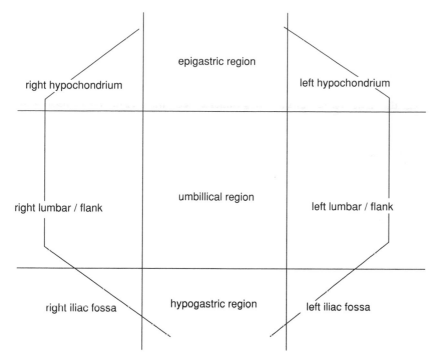

Figure 1.10. Abdominal examination.

GASTROINTESTINAL EXAMINATION

The approach is slightly different for this system. Auscultation comes after inspection followed by percussion and finally palpation.

INSPECTION

• Look for scars, striae, hernias, vascular changes, spider naevi, lesions, or rashes.
• Look for movement associated with peristalsis or pulsations.

AUSCULTATION

• Place the diaphragm of your stethoscope lightly on the abdomen.
• Listen for bowel sounds. Are they normal, increased, decreased, or absent?
• Listen for bruits over the renal arteries, iliac arteries, and aorta.

PERCUSSION

- Percuss in all nine areas.
- Percuss the liver:
  - ➢ begin in the right iliac fossa;
  - ➢ ensure the patient is breathing deeply;
  - ➢ use the radial border of the index finger to feel the liver edge;
  - ➢ move up 2 cm at a time;
  - ➢ assess its size, regularity, smoothness, and tenderness;
  - ➢ is it pulsatile?
  - ➢ confirm the lower border and define the upper border;
  - ➢ listen for an overlying bruit.

PALPATION

General Palpation

- Begin with light palpation.
- Look for areas of tenderness. Watch the patient's face.
- Look for voluntary or involuntary guarding.
- After light palpation continue with deep palpation.
- Identify abdominal masses or areas of deep tenderness.
- Check for rebound tenderness:
  - ➢ warn the patient what you are about to do;
  - ➢ press deeply on the abdomen with your hand;
  - ➢ after a moment, quickly release pressure;
  - ➢ if it hurts more when you release, the patient has rebound tenderness.
- Palpate the spleen:
  - ➢ use your left hand to lift the lower rib cage and flank;
  - ➢ press down just below the left costal margin with your right hand;
  - ➢ ask the patient to take a deep breath;
  - ➢ the spleen is not normally palpable on most individuals.
- Test for shifting dullness if ascites is suspected:
  - ➢ percuss the patient's abdomen to outline areas of dullness and tympany;
  - ➢ ask the patient to roll away from you;
  - ➢ percuss and again outline areas of dullness and tympany;
  - ➢ if the dullness has shifted to areas of prior tympany, the patient may have excess peritoneal fluid.
- If cholecystitis is suspected look for a positive Murphy's sign.
- Don't forget to perform a PR examination.
- Test for faecal occult blood (FOB).

NEUROLOGICAL EXAMINATION

In the acute setting of an MAU it may not be appropriate to undertake a full neu-rological examination. The need for this examination will depend on the presenting complaint of the patient. If a full neurological examination is required then use the following as a guide.

INSPECTION

- Always observe left to right symmetry.
- Consider central vs. peripheral deficits.
- Assess mental state using Hodkinson's (1972) abbreviated mental test score:
  - ➢ Ask the patient to answer the following questions. Score 1 point for each correct answer:

    1. age
    2. time (to nearest hour)
    3. an address for recall at the end of the test (42 West Street); ensure the patient has heard the address by asking them to repeat it after they are told it
    4. year
    5. name of hospital
    6. recognition of two persons (e.g. doctor and nurse)
    7. date of birth
    8. date of World War I
    9. name of present monarch
    10. count backwards from 20–1

A score of 7 or less is consistent with impaired brain function.

Cranial Nerve Examination

Observation

- Ptosis (III).
- Facial droop or asymmetry (VII).
- Hoarse voice (X).
- Articulation of words (V, VII, X, XII).
- Abnormal eye position (III, IV, VI).
- Abnormal or asymmetrical pupils (II, III).

I Olfactory

- Not normally tested.

II Optic

- Examine the optic fundi.
- Test visual acuity.
- Test pupillary reactions to light.
- Test pupillary reactions to accommodation:
  - ➢ hold your finger about 10 cm from the patient's nose;
  - ➢ ask them to alternate looking into the distance and at your finger;
  - ➢ observe the pupillary response in each eye.

III Oculomotor

- Observe for ptosis.
- Test extraocular movements.
- Stand or sit 3–6 feet in front of the patient.
- Ask the patient to follow your finger with their eyes without moving their head.
- Check gaze in the six cardinal directions using a cross or 'H' pattern.
- Pause during upward and lateral gaze to check for nystagmus.
- Check convergence by moving your finger towards the bridge of the patient's nose.
- Test pupillary reactions to light.

IV Trochlear

- Test extraocular movements (inward and down movement).

V Trigeminal

- Test temporal and masseter muscle strength:
    - ask patient to open their mouth and clench their teeth;
    - palpate the temporal and massetter muscles as they do this.
- Test the three divisions for pain sensation:
    - explain what you intend to do;
    - use a suitable sharp object to test the forehead, cheeks, and jaw on; both sides;
    - substitute a blunt object occasionally and ask the patient to report 'sharp' or 'dull'.
- If you find any abnormality then:
    - test the three divisions for temperature sensation with a tuning fork heated or cooled by water;
    - test the three divisions for sensation to light touch using a wisp of cotton.
- Test the corneal reflex:
    - ask the patient to look up and away;
    - from the other side, touch the cornea lightly with a fine wisp of cotton;
    - look for the normal blink reaction of both eyes;
    - repeat on the other side;
    - use of contact lenses may decrease this response.

VI Abducens

- Test extraocular movements (lateral movement).

VII Facial

- Observe for any facial droop or asymmetry.
- Ask patient to do the following, note any lag, weakness, or assymetry:
    - raise eyebrows
    - close both eyes to resistance

➤ smile
➤ frown
➤ show teeth
➤ puff out cheeks
➤ test the corneal reflex.

VIII Acoustic

- Screen hearing (if appropriate):
  ➤ face the patient and hold out your arms with your fingers near each ear;
  ➤ rub your fingers together on one side while moving the fingers noiselessly on the other;
  ➤ ask the patient to tell you when and on which side they hear the rubbing;
  ➤ increase intensity as needed and note any asymmetry.
- If abnormal, proceed with the Weber and Rinne tests.
- Test for lateralization:
  ➤ use a 512 Hz or 1024 Hz tuning fork;
  ➤ start the fork vibrating by tapping it on your opposite hand;
  ➤ place the base of the tuning fork firmly on top of the patient's head;
  ➤ ask the patient where the sound appears to be coming from (normally in the midline).
- Compare air and bone conduction – as above but utilising the following:
  ➤ place the base of the tuning fork against the mastoid bone behind the ear;
  ➤ when the patient no longer hears the sound, hold the end of the fork near the patient's ear (air conduction is normally greater than bone conduction).
- Vestibular function is not normally tested.

IX Glossopharyngeal and X Vagus

- Listen to the patient's voice, is it hoarse or nasal?
- Ask patient to swallow.
- Ask patient to say 'Ah'.
- Watch the movements of the soft palate and the pharynx.
- Test gag reflex (unconscious/uncooperative patient).
- Stimulate the back of the throat on each side.
- It is normal to gag after each stimulus.

XI Accessory

- From behind, look for atrophy or assymetry of the trapezius muscles.
- Ask patient to shrug shoulders against resistance.
- Ask patient to turn their head against resistance.
- Watch and palpate the sternomastoid muscle on the opposite side.

XII Hypoglossal

- Listen to the articulation of the patient's words.
- Observe the tongue as it lies in the mouth.

Grade out of 5	Muscle strength
0	No muscle movement
1	Visible muscle movement. No movement at joint
2	Movement at joint. No movement against gravity
3	Movement against gravity. Not against added resistance
4	Movement against resistance but less than normal
5	Normal strength

Figure 1.11. Muscle strength table.

- Ask patient to:
  - ➤ protrude tongue;
  - ➤ move tongue from side to side.

Motor

Observation: Look for Signs of:

- Involuntary movements.
- Muscle symmetry.
- Proximal and distal differences.
- Signs of atrophy.
- Pay particular attention to the hands, shoulders, and thighs.
- Observe gait if appropriate.

Muscle Tone

- Ask the patient to relax.
- Flex and extend the patient's fingers, wrist, and elbow.
- Flex and extend patient's ankle and knee.
- There is normally a small, continuous resistance to passive movement.
- Observe for decreased (flaccid) or increased (rigid/spastic) tone.

Muscle Strength

- Test strength by having the patient move against your resistance.
- Always compare one side to the other.
- Grade strength on a scale of 1–5.
- Test the following:
  - ➤ flexion and extension at the elbow;
  - ➤ extension at the wrist;

- ➤ squeeze two of your fingers as hard as possible;
- ➤ finger abduction;
- ➤ opposition of the thumb;
- ➤ flexion, extension, adduction and abduction at the hips;
- ➤ extension and flexion at the knee;
- ➤ dorsiflexion at the ankle;
- ➤ plantar flexion.
- • Assess pronator drift:
  - ➤ ask the patient to stand for 20–30 seconds with both arms straight forward, palms up and eyes closed;
  - ➤ instruct the patient to keep the arms still while you tap them briskly downward;
  - ➤ the patient will not be able to maintain extension and supination (and 'drift' into pronation) with upper motor neuron disease.

Coordination and Gait

- • Ask the patient to touch your index finger and their nose alternately several times.
- • Move your finger into different positions.
- • Hold your finger still so that the patient can touch it with one arm and finger outstretched.
- • Ask the patient to move their arm and return to your finger with their eyes closed.
- • Ask the patient to place one heel on the opposite knee and run it down the shin to the big toe. Repeat with the patient's eyes closed.
- • Test for Romberg's sign:
  - ➤ be prepared to catch the patient if they are unstable;
  - ➤ ask the patient to stand with their feet together and eyes closed for 5–10 seconds without support;
  - ➤ the test is said to be positive if the patient becomes unstable (indicating a vestibular or proprioceptive problem).
- • Assess the patient's gait if appropriate.

Reflexes

- • The patient must be relaxed and positioned properly before starting.
- • Reflex response depends on the force of your stimulus:
  - ➤ use no more force than you need to provoke a definite response.
- • If reflexes are hyperactive test for clonus:
  - ➤ support the knee in a partly flexed position;
  - ➤ with the patient relaxed, quickly dorsiflex the foot;
  - ➤ observe for rhythmic oscillations.
- • Assess subjective light touch.
- • Assess position sense:
  - ➤ grasp the patient's big toe and hold it away from the other toes to avoid friction;
  - ➤ show the patient 'up' and 'down';

➤ with the patient's eyes closed, ask the patient to identify the direction you move the toe;
➤ if position sense is impaired, move proximally to test the ankle joint;
➤ test the fingers in a similar fashion.

MUSCULOSKELETAL EXAMINATION

When examining the musculoskeletal system it is vital that you recall your anatomy. Think of the underlying anatomy as you undertake an examination. Always begin with inspection, palpation and range of motion.

Useful Hints

- When taking a history for an acute problem always enquire about the mechanism of injury.
- You can use SOCRATES.
- When taking a history for a chronic problem always inquire about:
  ➤ past injuries
  ➤ past treatments
  ➤ effect on function
  ➤ current symptoms.
- Signs of musculoskeletal disease are:
  ➤ pain
  ➤ redness (erythema)
  ➤ swelling
  ➤ increased warmth
  ➤ deformity
  ➤ loss of function.

INSPECTION

- Look for scars, rashes, or other lesions.
- Look for asymmetry, deformity, or atrophy.
- Always compare with the other side.

PALPATION

- Examine each major joint and muscle group in turn.
- Identify any areas of tenderness.
- Identify any areas of deformity.
- Always compare with the other side.

Range of Motion

When assessing range of motion, start by asking the patient to go through specific movements. If you detect anything abnormal proceed to a range of passive movements.

Active Movement

- Ask the patient to move each joint through a full range of motion.
- Note the degree and type (pain, weakness, etc.) of any limitations.
- Note any increased range of motion or instability.
- Always compare with the other side.
- Proceed to passive range of motion if abnormalities are found.

Passive Movement

- Ask the patient to relax and allow you to support the extremity to be examined.
- Gently move each joint through its full range of motion.
- Note the degree and type of any limitation (pain or mechanical).
- Always compare with the other side.

POST EXAMINATION

Now you have completed the examination explain to the patient what you think may be wrong, the investigations you wish to undertake and treatment.

CONCLUSION

The SOAPIE model and the medical model are, in reality, very similar. Whichever model you choose to use, be systematic in your approach, keep the patient informed, and document as you go along. Following these simple rules avoids confusion and ensures a comprehensive assessment of the patient.

REFERENCES

Bates B (1995) *A Guide to Physical Examination and History Taking*, 6th edn. Philadelphia: Lippincott.
Department of Health (2000) *The NHS Plan: A Plan for Investment, a Plan for Reform*. London: DoH.
Hodkinson HM (1972) Evaluation of a mental test score for assessment of mental impairment in the elderly *Age & Ageing* 1: 233–8.

Longmore M, Wilkinson I and Török E (2001) *Oxford Handbook of Clinical Medicine*, 5th edn. Oxford: Oxford University Press.

National Institute for Clinical Excellence (2004) *Chronic Obstructive Pulmonary Disease: Management of Chronic Obstructive Pulmonary Disease in Primary and Secondary Care*. Clinical Guideline 12. London: NICE.

Sprigings D and Chambers J (2001) *Acute Medicine: A Practical Guide to the Management of Medical Emergencies*, 3rd edn. Oxford: Blackwell Science.

Welsby P (2002) *Clinical History Taking and Examination*, 2nd edn. Edinburgh: Churchill Livingstone.

2 Emergencies

Clinical emergencies are commonplace in the medical assessment unit and acute medicine. Nurse practitioners need to possess the knowledge and skills to ensure safe and effective management of the emergency situation. It is highly recommended that practitioners undertake an Advanced Life Support Course in order to equip them for the emergency situation. The guidelines that follow are the current ones, based on a consensus of opinion recommended by the Resuscitation Council (UK) 2005.

ANAPHYLAXIS

DEFINITION

There are no universally accepted definitions of anaphylactic and anaphylactoid reactions.

Anaphyalxis is the term used for hypersensitivity reactions that are typically mediated by immunoglobulin E (IgE).

Anaphylactoid reactions are similar but do not depend on hypersensitivity.

The initial management of both types of reaction is the same and therefore the term anaphyalxis will be used throughout this section (Joint Council of Allergy, Asthma and Immunology 1998)

SYMPTOMS AND SIGNS

Anaphylactic reactions vary in their severity and the rate of onset and duration of symptoms. Some reactions can take several hours to manifest themselves and the symptoms may last for more than 24 hours.

The patient presenting with an anaphylactic reaction may have one or more of the following symptoms:

- angio-oedema
- urticaria
- dyspnoea
- hypotension – due to vasodilation and loss of plasma from blood compartment

Other symptoms include:

- rhinitis
- conjunctivitis

- abdominal pain
- vomiting
- diarrhoea
- some patients describe a sense of impending doom
- some may appear pale, others flushed

ASSESSMENT

A full history and examination should be undertaken at the earliest opportunity. A history of previous reactions as well as that of the current reaction is important.

It must be remembered that patients can and do die following anaphylactic reactions. It is therefore vital that prompt assessment is undertaken and any emergency situation dealt with safely and effectively.

Utilise an ABCDE approach to immediate assessment:

Airway

- Ensure patent airway.
- Nurse in recovery position if unconscious.
- Utilise guedel airway or nasopharyngeal airway if necessary.
- Consider intubation if unable to maintain airway.

Breathing

- Give high flow oxygen.
- Monitor oxygen saturations – aim to maintain above 92%.
- Monitor respiratory rate.
- Assist ventilation with bag valve mask if necessary.
- Measure Peak Expiratory Flow Rate (PEFR).
- Consider nebulised Salbutamol via oxygen.

Circulation

- Gain intravenous access.
- Ensure cardiac monitoring.
- Record ECG.
- Monitor blood pressure every five minutes initially.
- If hypotensive (BP <100/60) give sodium chloride 0.9% intravenously; patients may require 1–2 litres over a short period of time.
- Administer adrenaline 1:1,000 0.5 ml (500 mcg) IM.
- Repeat dose of adrenaline may be given in five minutes if no clinical improvement.

Disability

Assess using AVPU or Glasgow Coma Scale:

A – alert
V – responds to verbal commands
P – responds to pain
U – unresponsive

Exposure

• Look for rash and skin blisters.
• If unsure about cause – look for signs of insect bites, bee stings and snake bites.

LIFE-THREATENING FEATURES

• inspiratory stridor
• wheeze
• cyanosis
• pronounced tachycardia
• decreased capillary refill time

If the patient demonstrates any of these manifestations, call for help and administer adrenaline immediately, as per the anaphylaxis algorithm.
    Cardiopulmonary resuscitation (CPR) should be commenced if necessary.

CARDIO-RESPIRATORY ARREST

All health care workers need to be able to manage a patient in cardiac arrest. For most nurses this means the ability to confirm cardiac arrest and the undertaking of basic life support (BLS) until help arrives. As a nurse practitioner you are likely to form part of that 'help' and therefore need to be competent in the provision of Advanced Life Support (ALS). Most large hospitals run or have access to Resuscitation Council approved ALS courses and any nurse practitioner working in this acute speciality should undertake a course.
    The following guidelines were published jointly by the Resuscitation Council (UK) and the European Resuscitation Council in November 2005. They represent a consensus of opinion from Europe's experts in the field of resuscitation medicine. Evidence has been evaluated and the guidelines formed.
    An ABCDE approach is utilised when finding a patient collapsed.

• Confirm cardiac arrest – shake and shout.
• Call for help.

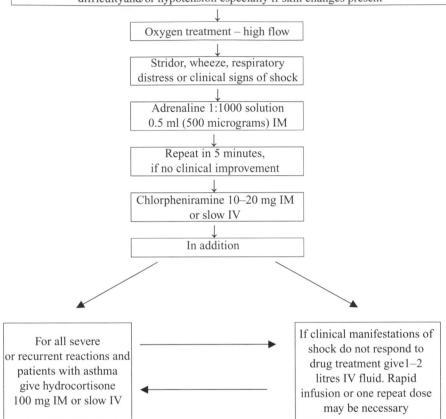

- An inhaled beta 2 agonist such as salbutamol may be used as an adjunctive measure if bronchospasm is severe and does not respond rapidly to other treatment.
- If profound shock judged immediately life threatening give CPR/ALS if necessary. Consider slow IV adrenaline 1:10,000 solution. This is hazardous and is recommended only for an experienced practitioner who can also obtain IV access without delay.
  Note the different strengths of adrenaline that may be required for IV use.
- If adults are treated with an adrenaline auto-injector, the 300 micrograms will usually be sufficient. A second dose may be required. Half doses of adrenaline may be safer for patients on amitriptylline, imipramine or beta blocker.
- A crystalloid may be safer than a colloid.

Figure 2.1. Anaphylaxis treatment algorithm. Reproduced with kind permission of the Resuscitation Council UK.

- If the patient is unresponsive – open airway, using head tilt and chin lift.
- Look in the mouth. If a foreign body is visible, attempt to remove it using suction or forceps.
- Keeping the airway open, look, listen and feel for no more than 10 seconds to determine if the patient is breathing normally.
- Assess the carotid pulse for no more than 10 seconds simultaneously.

If the patient has a pulse but is *not* breathing

- Ventilate the patient's lungs at a rate of 10 breaths per minute.
- Check for a pulse every 10 breaths.

If cardiac arrest is confirmed

- Commence CPR.
- Give 30 chest compressions followed by two ventilations.
- Hands should be placed over the lower half of the sternum. Compress the chest 4–5 cm at a rate of 100 compressions per minute.
- Maintain the airway using airway adjuncts – guedel airway, nasopharyngeal airway with pocket mask and supplemental oxygen or bag valve mask.
- Secure the airway with a laryngeal mask airway (LMA) or tracheal intubation if trained and skilled in this.
- Use an inspiratory time of one second and give enough volume to see the chest rise as in normal breathing.
- Once the patient's airway has been secured, continue chest compressions at a rate of 100 per minute uninterrupted, except for defibrillation or pulse checks. Ventilate the lungs at a rate of 10 breaths per minute.
- As soon as a defibrillator arrives, attach electrodes and assess rhythm.

SHOCKABLE RHYTHMS (VF AND PULSELESS VT)

- Attempt defibrillation by giving one shock (150–200 J biphasic or 360 J monophasic).
- Immediately resume chest compressions (30:2) without reassessing rhythm or checking for a pulse.
- Continue CPR for two minutes then pause briefly to check the monitor.
- If VF/VT persists, give a further shock (150–360 J biphasic, 360 J monophasic).
- Resume CPR immediately and continue for two minutes.
- Pause briefly to check the monitor.
- If VF/VT persists give adrenaline 1 mg IV followed immediately by a third shock (150–360 J biphasic, 360 J monophasic).
- Resume CPR immediately and continue for two minutes.
- Pause briefly to check the monitor

- If VF/VT persists give amiodarone 300 mg IV followed immediately by a fourth shock (150–360 J biphasic, 360 J monophasic).
- Resume CPR immediately and continue for two minutes.
- Give adrenaline 1 mg before alternate shocks (every 3–5 minutes).
- Give a further shock after every two-minute period of CPR and confirming VF/VT persists.
- If organised electrical activity is seen during the brief pause in compressions, check for a pulse.
- If no pulse is present, continue CPR and switch to the non-shockable algorithm.
- If asystole is seen, continue CPR and switch to the non-shockable algorithm.

PRECORDIAL THUMP

- Consider giving a precordial thump immediately after cardiac arrest is confirmed if the arrest was witnessed and monitored.
- Use the ulnar edge of a tightly clenched fist.
- Deliver a sharp impact to the lower half of the sternum from a height of about 20 cm.
- Retract the fist immediately.

NON-SHOCKABLE RHYTHM – PULSELESS ELECTRICAL ACTIVITY (PEA)

- Commence CPR (30:2).
- Give adrenaline 1 mg IV as soon as IV access is achieved.
- Continue CPR (30:2) until the airway is secured then continue chest compressions without pausing during ventilation.
- Recheck the rhythm after two minutes.
- Give further adrenaline 1 mg IV every 3–5 minutes.
- If the ECG changes and organised electrical activity is seen, check for a pulse.
- If a pulse is present start post resuscitation care.
- If no pulse is present continue CPR.
- Recheck the rhythm every two minutes.
- Give further adrenaline 1 mg IV every 3–5 minutes (alternate loops).

NON-SHOCKABLE RHYTHM – ASYSTOLE AND SLOW PEA (RATE <60 MIN)

- Start CPR 30:2.
- Without stopping CPR check that the leads are attached correctly.
- Give adrenaline 1 mg IV as soon as IV access is obtained.
- Give atropine 3 mg IV (once only).
- Continue CPR (30:2) until the airway is secured then continue chest compressions without pausing during ventilation.

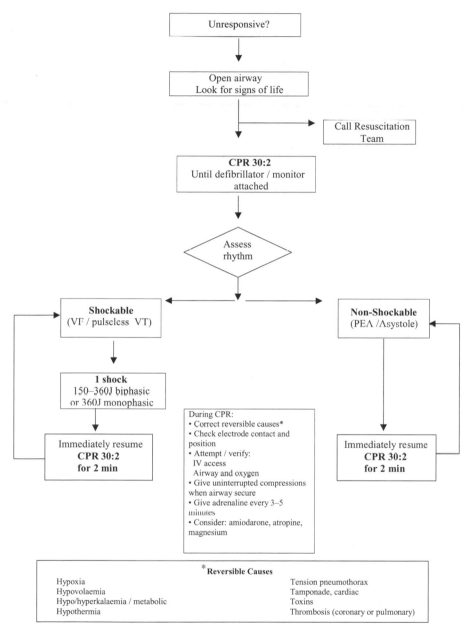

Figure 2.2. The universal ALS algorithm. Reproduced with kind permission of the Resuscitation Council UK.

- Recheck the rhythm after two minutes.
- Give further adrenaline 1 mg IV every 3–5 minutes.
- If VF/VT occurs change to the shockable algorithm.
- Do not be tempted to treat asystole as fine VF. Always treat as a non-shockable rhythm.

REVERSIBLE CAUSES – THE FOUR 'H's AND THE FOUR 'T's

During any cardiac arrest it is important to look for potential causes or aggravating factors for which specific treatments exist. The Resuscitation Council calls these the four 'H's and the four 'T's for ease of recall. They are:

- hypoxia
- hypovolaemia
- hyperkalaemia, hypokalaemia, hypocalcaemia, acidaemia and other metabolic disturbances
- hypothermia

- tension pneumothorax
- tamponade
- toxic substances
- thromboembolism (pulmonary embolus / coronary thrombosis)

Hypoxia

- Ensure adequate ventilation with 100% oxygen.
- Ensure adequate chest rise.
- Listen for bilateral breath sounds.
- If intubated ensure correct position of tracheal tube.

Hypovolaemia

- Expose the patient – look for signs of bleeding/ fluid loss.
- Gain multiple IV access.
- Restore intravascular volume with IV fluid given rapidly – the patient is in cardiac arrest – give whatever fluid is available.
- Urgent referral to the surgeons may be required if cardiac output is returned.

Hyperkalaemia

- During cardiac arrest there is no point in obtaining venous blood samples.
- Ascertain the most recent biochemical test results.
- Ask if the patient has had a recent ECG – look for peaked T waves suggesting hyperkalaemia.

- Look at the drug chart – are they taking any medication that may cause a metabolic disturbance?
- Is there any history which may lead you to suspect a metabolic disturbance (e.g. renal failure)?
- Intravenous calcium chloride can be given in the presence of hyperkalaemia, hypocalcaemia and calcium channel blocking drug overdose.

Hypothermia

Hypothermia is defined as the core body temperature falling below 35 °C. It can be difficult to distinguish between death and hypothermia.

- Mild hypothermia – 35–32 °C.
- Moderate hypothermia – 32–30 °C.
- Severe hypothermia – less than 30 °C.

Always check for a pulse and respiratory effort for one minute if patient is hypothermic.

- Movement may precipitate arrhythmias.
- Chest stiffness may make ventilation and compressions difficult.
- Defibrillation may not be effective when core body temperature is <30 °C – consider delaying until temperature >30 °C.
- Resuscitation may be prolonged – the adage being that the patient isn't dead until they are warm and dead.
- Slowly re-warm.
- Use warmed fluids.
- Consider gastric and bladder lavage with warmed fluids.
- If available consider utilisation of bypass and Extra Corporeal Membrane Oxygenation (ECMO).

Tension Pneumothorax

The diagnosis is made clinically. Features are:

- Diminished breath sounds on the affected side.
- Hyperresonance on the affected side.
- Tracheal deviation to the contralateral side.

Treatment is by emergency decompression of the tension.

- Insert a large bore canuala into the second intercostal space in the midclavicular line on the affected side.
- If successful you will hear a hiss of air.
- After successful resuscitation a chest drain must be inserted.

Tamponade

Tamponade is often difficult to diagnose in the cardiac arrest situation. The usual signs of tamponade are distended neck veins and hypotension. These are absent during cardiac arrest. A tamponade should be suspected if there is a history of chest trauma. Treatment is needle pericardiocentesis, which requires expert assistance.

Toxic Substances

History may lead you to suspect that toxic substances are a cause of cardiac arrest. If you know what the toxin is give the antidote. If you are unsure what the antidote is, help can be found by ringing your local poisons unit or by accessing Toxbase (www.spib.axl.co.uk – see Chapter 3 for more information).

Some common toxins and their antidotes are:

- paracetamol – N-acetylcysteine
- digoxin – digoxin specific FAB antibodies
- benzodiazepines – flumazenil
- opioids – naloxone
- tricyclics – consider administering sodium bicarbonate intravenously
- beta blockers – glucagon

Thromboembolism

The most common cause is pulmonary embolism.

- Consider thrombolysis during cardiac arrest if this is suspected as the cause.

ETHICAL ISSUES

BREAKING BAD NEWS

Following an unsuccessful resuscitation, relatives need to be informed. As the nurse practitioner this may fall to you. What you say to the relative will stay with them forever, so it is vital that it is done well and correctly.

It is likely that while the resuscitation attempt has been ongoing, another member of staff will have contacted the relatives if they were not already present. It is good practice when you are summoned to a cardiac arrest to ensure someone is contacting the relatives.

If relatives have not already been contacted, do so immediately. This will usually be by phone. When the phone is answered, introduce yourself but clarify who you are speaking to. For example, 'Is that Mrs Jones, the wife of Mr William Jones?'

Some practitioners do not like to break bad news over the telephone, preferring to inform the relative that their loved one is seriously ill and then ask them to come to the hospital. However, that can then make it difficult to answer questions relatives may have about the death. Frequently relatives want to know exactly when their loved one died and they may be angry when informed that they were already dead before they were asked to come to the hospital, having preferred to have been informed over the telephone. There is no right or wrong answer to this. The circumstances surrounding every individual resuscitation are unique, and each situation should be dealt with accordingly. Other staff on the unit may know that the relative is elderly and on their own at home with no other family. In this situation it may be appropriate to say that their loved one is seriously ill and ask them to come to the hospital where the news can be imparted gently and they can be supported by staff. In another situation the relative may be hundreds of miles away and they are going to take several hours to get to their loved one. It may be more appropriate to inform them over the telephone. As a practitioner you must utilise your expertise to make a decision or advise others on the most appropriate course of action.

Never lie to a relative. If they ask you over the telephone you must be honest and tell them what has occurred.

Some general rules when breaking bad news are:

- Ensure you have somewhere quiet, private and free from interruptions to talk to relatives.
- Confirm that you are talking to the correct relatives.
- Always sit at the same height as the relatives.
- Do not give the impression you are busy or in a hurry.
- Use the words 'dead' or 'died'. Do not leave room for doubt.
- Don't be afraid of long pauses. Relatives need time to assimilate what they have been told.
- Touching may be appropriate.
- Be prepared for a variety of reactions. Everyone responds to bad news differently.
- Ask relatives if they have any questions.
- Make sure you know what local policies are for collecting belongings, death certificates and registering the death.
- Allow the relatives the opportunity to view their loved one if they so wish.

DO NOT ATTEMPT RESUSCITATION ORDERS (DNAR)

The phrase 'do not attempt resuscitation' means that in the event of a cardiac or respiratory arrest CPR should not be attempted. It does not mean that all treatment should be stopped.

DNAR decisions should only be made by the most senior clinician responsible for the patient. This is usually the consultant physician but in their absence this may be delegated to a specialist registrar. It is important that you familiarise yourself with your local policy regarding this decision-making process. However, it is likely that you will be called upon to help in this decision-making process.

If possible resuscitation should be discussed with the patient. This conversation should ascertain what the patient's wishes are regarding resuscitation. The patient's wishes should prevail.

If the patient is unable to make a balanced judgement or is too ill the senior clinician should discuss resuscitation with next of kin and close relatives. While their opinion should be taken into account and may influence the decision-making process it must be made clear to them that the ultimate decision remains with the senior clinician.

Decisions should be documented clearly in the medical notes along with the clinical justification, who the matter was discussed with and when or if the decision should be reviewed. This should be signed and dated, and the clinician's name and designation clearly written in the notes. Again, individual hospitals will have local policies and you should familiarise yourself with these.

Once the decision has been made, all staff caring for the patient must be made aware of the decision and this must also be communicated to the patient if possible and the patient's relatives.

FAMILY PRESENCE DURING RESUSCITATION

Family member presence during resuscitation is common practice in paediatrics. In the adult health care arena this is a relatively new concept. Small studies have shown that family members benefit and would like to be present during resuscitation attempts (Hanson and Strawser 1992; Chalk 1995; Robinson et al. 1998; Royal College of Nursing 2002). The benefits shown are of knowing that everything was done for their loved one and coming to terms with the death better. It must be emphasised that these studies were small and whether or not these benefits are sustained over a long period of time is as yet unknown.

In 2002 the RCN and BMA issued joint guidelines to enable this practice to occur and in this context research suggests that the following should be ensured:

- If a family member wishes to be present, this should be accommodated. Lack of space and team leader reluctance are not reasons for not allowing them to be present.
- The family member should not be made to feel as if they are in the way or intruding.
- Ensure that an experienced member of staff, who can explain to the relative what is happening, accompanies them at all times.
- Before the relative goes into the area, ensure that they know what to expect – explain to them what they will see, hear and smell.
- Ensure that the relative understands it is their choice whether they stay or go and they can come and go as they wish.
- The accompanying nurse must remain with the relative at all times and must not get involved in the resuscitation attempt.
- The accompanying nurse must ensure that the relative remains safe at all times – special care must be taken during defibrillation.
- Allow the relative to stand close to their loved one but in a position where they will not interrupt the resuscitation effort.

- Allow the relative to touch their loved one and talk to them if they so wish.
- If the family member wishes to leave the resuscitation attempt the accompanying nurse must go with them and ensure they have a quiet, private place to wait.
- If a decision to stop the resuscitation attempt is made this should be made in the usual way by the team leader in conjunction with the rest of the team. This decision must then be explained to the family member.
- The family member should be allowed time with their loved one. It may be appropriate to ask if they wish to remain with them immediately after the resuscitation is stopped or to have some quiet time and return later.
- The team leader must talk to the family after the event in the same way as they would if the family had not been present during resuscitation.
- The family must be allowed the opportunity to ask questions.
- Should family members disrupt the resuscitation attempt they must be removed to a quiet area by the accompanying nurse who must remain with them at all times.

REFERENCES

Chalk A (1995) Should relatives be present in the resuscitation room? *Accident and Emergency Nursing* 3(2): 58–61.

Hanson C and Strawser D (1992) Family presence during cardiopulmonary resuscitation: Foote Hospital Emergency Department's nine year perspective study. *Journal of Emergency Nursing* 18(2): 104–6.

Joint Council of Allergy, Asthma and Immunology (1998) The diagnosis and management of anaphylaxis. *Journal of Allergy and Clinical Immunology* 101: 465–528.

Resuscitation Council (UK) (2005) *Resuscitation Guidelines 2005*, ed. A Handley. London: Resuscitation Council.

Robinson SM, Mackenzie-Ross S, Campbell Hewson GL, Egleston CV and Prevost AT (1998) Psychological effects of witnessed resuscitation on bereaved relatives. *The Lancet* 352(9128): 614–17.

Royal College of Nursing (2002) *Witnessing Resuscitation: Guidance for Nursing Staff*. London: RCN Publications.

3   Acute Poisoning and Drug Overdose

DELIBERATE SELF-HARM

Deliberate self-harm is sadly seen on a daily basis in medical assessment units. In today's society practitioners need to be able to manage the act of deliberate self-harm with drugs such as paracetamol, aspirin and tricyclic antidepressants but also alcohol and illicit substances.

DEFINITION

Poisoning is defined as the chemical injury to organs of the body or a chemically induced disturbance of the function of the bodies systems.

INCIDENCE

Every year in the United Kingdom there are 300,000 cases of poisoning; 100,000 of these will be admitted to hospital. Between 3,500 and 4,000 people die every year as a result of poisoning (Office for National Statistics 2005).

SYMPTOMS AND SIGNS

Always consider acute poisoning / drug overdose in any unconscious adult (Resuscitation Council UK 2005).

The drug history may be unreliable. Always question witnesses / family members. Ask about the patient's own drugs, access to other drugs and any empty packets or bottles found at the scene of the overdose. The attending paramedics are a good source of information. Try and identify the likely poison as soon as possible.

Common features relating to specific drugs are:

- A depressed respiratory drive – suggests a centrally acting drug may have been taken.
- Skin blisters – suggest barbiturates or tricyclics may have been ingested.
- Hypothermia – can occur after barbiturate overdose or if patient has been exposed in an unconscious state.
- Look for needle marks in the arms and pinpoint pupils – suggestive of opioid overdose.

ASSESSMENT

Follow an ABCDE approach to assessment and treatment.

Airway

- Ensure patent airway.
- Nurse in recovery position if unconscious.
- Utilise guedel airway or nasopharyngeal airway if necessary.
- Consider intubation if unable to maintain airway.
- Remember there is a high risk of aspiration in the unconscious patient following overdose and therefore the airway can be compromised at a later stage even if it isn't now.

Breathing

- Give high flow oxygen if unconscious – unless paraquat poisoning is suspected as this can exacerbate pulmonary injury.
- Monitor oxygen saturations.
- Monitor respiratory rate.
- Assist ventilation with bag valve mask if necessary.
- If respiratory rate <12 per minute give naloxone 800 mcg – 2 mg IV to a maximum of 10 mg every two minutes until respiratory rate is within normal limits.
- *Remember* – the half life of naloxone is shorter than that of opiates so further doses may be required.

Circulation

- Gain intravenous access.
- Ensure cardiac monitoring.
- Record ECG.
- Monitor blood pressure at least every half hour.
- If hypotensive – BP <100/60, give sodium chloride 0.9% intravenously.
- If hypotension does not respond to intravenous fluids, a central line should be considered.
- Summon medical assistance.

Disability

Assess using AVPU or Glasgow Coma Scale.

Exposure

Look for needle marks, skin blisters, empty packets, undigested tablets.

Eye Opening	E
spontaneous	4
to speech	3
to pain	2
no response	1
Best Motor Response	**M**
obeys commands	6
localising pain	5
withdrawal from pain	4
flexion to pain	3
extension to pain	2
no motor response	1
Best Verbal Response	**V**
orientated	5
confused	4
inappropriate words	3
incomprehensible sounds	2
no response	1

Scoring

$E + M + V = 3 - 15$

A GCS of 13 or higher correlates with mild brain injury
9–12 is a moderate injury
8 or less is a severe brain injury

Figure 3.1. The Glasgow Coma Scale. *Source:* Reprinted from the *Lancet* (ii) Teasdale G and Jennett B (1974) The Glasgow Coma Scale, pp. 81–3. Reproduced with kind permission of Elsevier.

LIFE-THREATENING FEATURES

- Coma – defined as:
  - ➤ not opening eyes
  - ➤ not obeying commands
  - ➤ not uttering understandable words – assess Glasgow Coma Scale (GCS) (Teasdale and Jennett 1974).
- Cyanosis – clinical observation – assess for peripheral and central cyanosis.
- Hypotension – as already discussed give sodium chloride 0.9% IV and consider central line.
- Paralytic ileus – a functional obstruction due to reduced bowel motility. There is often no abdominal pain but bowel sounds are absent. Listen for bowel sounds.
- If the patient has any life-threatening features summon help immediately.

IMMEDIATE INVESTIGATIONS

- Obtain venous blood samples for urea and electrolytes (U&E), paracetamol levels, liver function tests (LFTs) and international normalising ratio (INR).
- Obtain arterial blood gases.

- Ensure samples of blood and urine are saved as they may be needed for further toxicology screening.
- Obtain an ECG and chest x-ray.

IMMEDIATE MANAGEMENT

You should have already followed the ABC approach.

- If not already done ensure high-flow oxygen (unless paraquat poisoning).
- Gain intravenous access.
- Obtain required blood samples (see above).
- Record an ECG.
- Assess GCS.
- Record temperature, pulse, blood pressure, respiratory rate and oxygen saturations.
- If decreased level of consciousness – insert urinary catheter.
- If you can prescribe or have a Patient Group Direction (PGD – see Chapter 13) in place and patient is hypotensive, give sodium chloride 0.9% intravenously.
- Identify the poison.
- If acutely unwell or you are unsure – get help.
- Consider gastric lavage – this should only be undertaken if the patient's airway can be protected and if they have ingested a life-threatening amount of a drug or toxic substance within the last hour. Realistically this is usually done in emergency departments and not in the MAU setting; therefore most nurse practitioners working in MAU are not likely to be trained in this procedure. However, if you are competent to perform this, it should be considered. Do not undertake gastric lavage if the patient has ingested corrosive substances.
- If you know what the poison is and it has a specific antidote if you can prescribe it or if you have a PGD (Chapter 13) then give the antidote. If you cannot, however frustrating it may be, find someone who can prescribe it. Administer the antidote and monitor its effect.
- Make sure you keep the patient (if conscious) informed of what you are doing and gain consent for investigation and treatment.
- If the patient is conscious, ascertain if they want anyone contacting about their admission and what they want next of kin to be told / not told
- If the patient is unconscious it is likely that a family member or friend has been the person that has found them and summoned help. They are going to be a vital source of information in helping identify the likely poison. However, the patient still has a right to confidentiality, so only disclose information that is necessary in order for you to ensure patient safety and aid recovery of the patient.
- All patients will require assessment by psychiatric services when medically fit for discharge.

Specific Poisons

PARACETAMOL OVERDOSE

Paracetamol is probably one of the most common drugs ingested during an act of deliberate self-harm. It is cheap and readily available. Sadly, the consequences of overdose can be fatal. According to the Office for National Statistics, in 2003 there were 86 deaths in England and Wales as a result of paracetamol overdose. The figure has improved since the late 1990s when there were 150 deaths per year. This is probably due to the restrictions on pack sizes which was enforced by the Medicines Control Agency in 1998.

RISK OF TOXICITY

If the patient has ingested less than 150 mg per kg of body weight of paracetamol it is unlikely that serious toxicity will occur, unless they have risk factors (Toxbase 2005).

Risk factors are:

- patients on long-term treatment with carbamazepine, phenobarbitone, phenytoin, rifampicin or St John's wort;
- patients who frequently consume alcohol in excess of the recommended amounts or have taken alcohol in combination with the paracetamol overdose;
- patients who are likely to be glutathione deplete, e.g. suffering from eating disorders or cystic fibrosis.

RISK OF LIVER DAMAGE – PEAK ALT 1,000 IU/LITRE

If the patient has ingested:

- less than 150 mg per kg body weight – liver damage unlikely
- more than 250 mg per kg body weight – liver damage likely
- more than 12 grams in total – potentially fatal

FEATURES

- Nausea and vomiting are extremely common.
- In patients who have very high paracetamol plasma concentrations, coma and severe metabolic acidosis can occur.
- 2–3 days after ingestion features of hepatic necrosis may occur:
  - ➤ right subcostal pain and tenderness
  - ➤ nausea and vomiting
  - ➤ jaundice.

Features of incipient renal failure are:

- loin pain
- haematuria
- proteinuria

ASSESSMENT AND INVESTIGATION SPECIFIC TO PARCETAMOL OVERDOSE

- Use an ABC approach to assessment – as documented above.
- Ascertain how much paracetamol was taken.
- What time was it taken?
- Was it all taken at once or was the overdose staggered? (See management of staggered overdose.)
- Were any other tablets or substances taken at the same time? It is not uncommon for people to take multiple drugs during an act of self-harm.
- Was alcohol taken at the same time?
- If alcohol was taken, how much was consumed?
- Ascertain if the patient has any specific risk factors as detailed previously.
- Obtain venous blood for paracetamol levels at least four hours after ingestion as peak plasma concentration will not occur before this time.
- Monitor LFTs, INR and U&E.
- Obtain arterial blood gases to monitor pH levels.

TREATMENT

- Treatment is with N-acetylcysteine (Parvolex®).
- Treatment doses are based on body weight.
- The need to deliver treatment is based on the plasma paracetamol concentration according to the nomogram (reproduced by kind permission of Alun Hutchings).
- Patients who have delayed in presenting following paracetamol overdose, or who have taken a staggered overdose, do not follow this guideline. Treatment in these circumstances is discussed later.
- As an independent nurse prescriber you can prescribe Parvolex® (Department of Health, May 2005). If you are not an independent prescriber, utilise a PGD or obtain the assistance of medical staff to prescribe treatment.
- Each ampoule of Parvolex contains 2 grams of N-acetylcysteine.

STAGGERED OVERDOSE OR DELAYED PRESENTATION

Patients who present more than 24 hours after ingesting paracetamol or who have taken paracetamol over a prolonged period of time (24 hours) can be challenging to manage as paracetamol levels cannot be interpreted and the nomogram cannot be utilised.

	Parvolex	Volume of 5% dextrose for dilution	
Dose	mg/kg body weight		Duration of infusion
1	150	200 mls	15 minutes
2	50	500 mls	4 hours
3	100	1000 mls	16 hours

Figure 3.2. Parvolex doses – give in sequence.

For any patient who presents and is in this category:

- Utilise an ABC approach.
- Obtain venous blood sample for LFTs, INR and U&E.
- Cannulate.
- Commence N-acetylcyseine immediately as in Figure 3.2.
- Continue Parvolex® for 24 hours after the last paracetamol was ingested.
- If LFTs and INR are within normal limits 24 hours after the last paracetamol dose was ingested, it is unlikely that significant toxicity has occurred and Parvolex® can be stopped.
- Patients who have delayed in presentation or taken a staggered overdose do not conform to the normal rules for paracetamol overdose. If in doubt contact your local poisons unit for advice.

ADVERSE REACTIONS TO N-ACETYLCYSTEINE

15% of patients given IV Parvolex® suffer an adverse reaction to it. Adverse reactions usually occur in the first 30 minutes of its administration as large amounts of the drug are being given rapidly. Common signs and symptoms of an adverse reaction are:

- nausea and vomiting
- flushing
- urticarial rash

A severe reaction requiring immediate life-saving treatment is rare but the patient may develop:

- angioedema
- tachycardia and hypotension
- bronchospasm
- respiratory depression
- collapse

In very severe cases:

- renal failure
- disseminated intravascular coagulation (DIC)

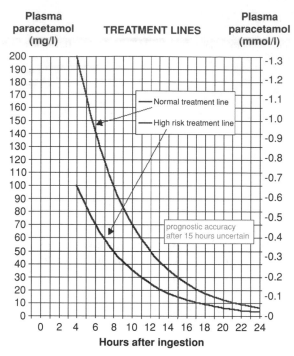

Figure 3.3. Reproduced by kind permission of Dr Alun Hutchings, WCM, Toxicology and Therapeutics Centre.

MANAGEMENT OF AN ADVERSE REACTION

- Stop the infusion – this is usually all that is required.
- If necessary give chlorpheniramine 4 mg orally or IV.
- If the reaction is severe follow an ABC approach and summon help immediately.
- If the reaction is severe give hydrocortisone 100 mg IV. Later this can be followed by a seven-day course of Prednisolone 30 mg once daily.
- If bronchospasm is severe, give high-flow oxygen and salbutamol 5 mg nebuliser.
- If you are not an independent prescriber you can give high-flow oxygen and a salbutamol nebuliser as emergency treatment under the Nursing and Midwifery Council Code of Professional Conduct (2002) for the purpose of saving life.
- Once the reaction has settled, recommence the Parvolex® infusion at a rate of 50 mg/kg body weight over four hours.
- It is highly unlikely that a further reaction will occur.

ASPIRIN OVERDOSE

Like paracetamol, aspirin overdose is sadly common. Aspirin is a non-steroidal anti-inflammatory which is readily available in most shops and supermarkets. While there is some media attention about the dangers of taking too many paracetamol tablets aspirin does not seem to attract the same degree of attention. Incidences of aspirin overdose are, like paracetamol, on the decline since the inception of legislation in 1998 governing the number of tablets in a packet and the number of packets that can be sold at any one time. However, it is still seen all too frequently in the medical assessment unit.

RISK OF TOXICITY

The risk of toxicity is determined by the amount of aspirin in milligrams ingested per kilogram of body weight (Toxbase 2003). If the patient has ingested:

- >120 mg per kg body weight – risk of toxicity is mild
- >250 mg per kg body weight – risk of toxicity is moderate
- 500 mg per kg body weight or more – toxicity is likely to be severe, possibly fatal.

FEATURES

Common features associated with aspirin overdose are:

- nausea and vomiting
- dehydration
- tinnitus
- vertigo
- deafness
- sweating
- warm extremities with bounding pulse
- increased respiratory rate with hyperventilation
- most patients will have some degree of acid-base disturbance

The common acid-base disturbance seen in aspirin overdose are:

- a mixed respiratory alkalosis
- a metabolic acidosis
- a normal or high pH

There are certain features of aspirin overdose that are uncommon but may occur and the practitioner should be aware of. These are:

- haematemesis
- hyperpyrexia
- hypoglycaemia
- thrombocytopoenia
- increased INR / APTT
- intravascular coagulation
- renal failure
- non-cardiac pulmonary oedema

- confusion and disorientation
- convulsions
- coma

ASSESSMENT OF SEVERITY

- Obtain venous blood sample for salicylate plasma concentration. The severity of toxicity cannot be assessed on the plasma salicylate level alone but aids assessment.
- Salicylate toxicity is usually associated with plasma concentrations >350 mg/l (Toxbase 2005).
- Most adult deaths occur in patients whose plasma concentration exceeds 700 mg/l (Toxbase 2005).

Severe poisoning is indicated if the patient has:

- confusion
- impaired consciousness
- metabolic acidosis
- high salicylate plasma concentration

Risk factors for death are:

- patient over 70 years of age
- central nervous system features
- acidosis
- hyperpyrexia
- late presentation following ingestion
- pulmonary oedema
- plasma salicylate concentration >700 mg/L

ASSESSMENT AND INVESTIGATION SPECIFIC TO ASPIRIN OVERDOSE

- Obtain salicylate levels at least two hours after ingestion as peak plasma concentrations will not occur before this time.
- Repeat sample two hours after first sample.
- Obtain arterial blood gases.
- Obtain venous blood for U&E, INR, APTT and blood glucose.
- If the patient shows signs of severe toxicity, summon medical assistance.

TREATMENT

- Give 50 grams of activated charcoal if more than 120 mg/kg body weight has been ingested in the last hour.
- If the serum potassium is within normal range and the patient has a metabolic acidosis, this can be corrected using intravenous sodium bicarbonate to enhance urinary salicylate excretion.

- Sodium bicarbonate dose is:
  - ➢ 1.5 litres of 1.26% sodium bicarbonate over two hours.
  - ➢ alternatively give 225 mls of 8.4% sodium bicarbonate over two hours.
- If serum potassium is low this must be corrected before giving sodium bicarbonate.
- Summon medical assistance.
- Forced diuresis should not be utilised as it does not enhance salicylate excretion and can cause pulmonary oedema.

There is a role for haemodialysis in patients with severe aspirin toxicity. Advice should be sought from intensive care and the renal team in the following circumstances:

- plasma concentrations >700 mg/l
- renal failure
- congestive cardiac failure
- non-cardiogenic pulmonary oedema
- convulsions
- central nervous system effects that do not resolve on correction of the acid base balance
- severe metabolic acidosis

TRICYCLIC ANTIDEPRESSANT OVERDOSE

Tricyclic antidepressants are used by many people in today's society. Overdose is relatively common.

RISK OF TOXICITY

- First-generation tricyclic antidepressants are more likely to cause lethal toxicity than the newer second-generation drugs (Toxbase 2005).
- First-generation drugs include amitriptyline and impramine.
- Second-generation drugs include lofepramine.
- There is a risk of severe toxicity in patients who have taken more than 4 mg per kilogram body weight of any tricyclic antidepressant.

FEATURES

Patients who have taken tricyclic antidepressants in overdose are likely to present with the following symptoms:

- dry mouth
- blurred vision
- sinus tachycardia
- nystagmus
- urinary retention

- muscle twitching
- agitation
- hallucinations

Severe toxicity can lead to:

- coma
- respiratory depression and hypoxia
- metabolic acidosis
- hypothermia
- skin blistering
- rhabdomyolosis
- prolongation of the QRS complex

ASSESSMENT AND INVESTIGATION SPECIFIC TO TRICYCLIC ANTIDEPRESSANT OVERDOSE

- Obtain venous blood sample for U&E.
- Obtain arterial blood gases to monitor acid-base balance.
- Record ECG to measure QRS length.
- Cardiac monitoring for 24 hours after ingestion.
- Monitor blood pressure as there is a risk of hypotension.
- Record temperature.
- Monitor urine output.

TREATMENT

- In patients who have taken a potentially serious overdose and who present within one hour of ingestion give 50 grams of activated charcoal orally.
- If the patient demonstrates signs of central nervous system toxicity, a further dose of activated charcoal can be given after two hours.
- If a sustained release preparation has been taken, give 50 grams of activated charcoal every four hours to a total of 220 grams.
- Give high flow oxygen if hypoxic.
- Correct metabolic acidosis (pH <7.2) if accompanied by hypotension (systolic BP <100 mmHg).
- Use 1.26% sodium bicarbonate (150 mmol/l) and give 50 mmols over 30 minutes.
- Repeat arterial blood gases after 30 minutes and give a further 50 mmols of sodium bicarbonate if acidosis persists
- Correct hypotension with 500 mls of gelofusine over 1 hour.
- If hypotension is unresponsive to gelofusine, give glucagon 1 mg every three minutes.
- If hypotension responds to glucagon, sustain this response by commencing an intravenous infusion of 2–4 mg an hour.

- If convulsions occur, treat them with diazepam intravenously. Give 5–20 mg no faster than 5 mg per minute.
- If diazepam cannot be used, give lorazepam 4 mg over two minutes into a large vein.
- Manage hypothermia by slowly re-warming no faster than 1 °C per hour.
- Manage any skin blisters as burns.
- Recovery following severe toxicity may be marked by profound agitation and florid visual and auditory hallucinations and should be treated with oral diazepam. Doses as high as 20–30 mg every two hours may be required.
- Monitor urine output and catheterise if urinary retention occurs.
- If cardiac arrest occurs, resuscitation should be prolonged as the cardiotoxic effects of tricyclic overdose diminish with time.

HEROIN OVERDOSE

TOXICITY

Toxicity is due to the opioid effects of heroin administration. A fatal overdose can occur after ingestion of approximately 200 mg of heroin (Toxbase 2000).

FEATURES

Common features of heroin overdose are:

- nausea and vomiting
- respiratory depression
- cyanosis
- pin point pupils

Severe features are:

- hypotension
- tachycardia
- hallucinations
- respiratory arrest

ASSESSMENT AND INVESTIGATION OF HEROIN OVERDOSE

- Utilise an ABC approach.
- Obtain venous blood samples for U&E, INR, LFTs and toxicology.
- Ensure cardiac monitoring.
- Obtain an ECG.
- Obtain arterial blood gases.
- Inspect for injection sites.

TREATMENT

If the Patient is Conscious

- If the patient presents within 1 hour of injecting / ingesting heroin and they can protect their own airway safely, give 50 grams of activated charcoal.
- Monitor respirations and blood pressure for a minimum of four hours after the overdose but for longer if the preparation taken was sustained release.

If the Patient is Unconscious

- Use the ABC approach and commence cardiopulmonary resuscitation (CPR) if necessary.
- Maintain airway using adjuncts if necessary.
- Nurse in the recovery position.
- Give high-flow oxygen.
- Monitor blood pressure, pulse, respiratory rate and oxygen saturations.
- Give naloxone (narcan) if respiratory rate <12 per minute. Administer 0.4–2 mg intravenously and repeat at two-minute intervals to a maximum of 10 mg if there is no response.
- The half life of naloxone is shorter than that of heroin and so beware that symptoms of heroin overdose may recur.
- If IV access is not possible, naloxone may be given intramuscularly.
- If repeated stat doses are required, an infusion can be administered. Set up an infusion of 10 mg naloxone made up to 50 mls with 5% dextrose. The initial rate at which the infusion should run is 60% of the total amount in milligrams of the stat doses required during the first hour of treatment.
- The patient must be observed for at least six hours after the last dose of naloxone was administered.

ALCOHOL OVERDOSE

Traditionally alcohol overdose is seen in emergency departments but as MAUs increase their capacity it is becoming the remit of these units to deal with this presenting problem. In order to understand toxicity it is important that practitioners have insight into the amount of alcohol contained in individual servings (see Figure 3.4).

Beverage	Approximate alcohol by volume	Alcohol (mg/ml)	Serving	Alcohol (g) per serving
Spirits	40%	316	25 ml / 35 ml	7.9/11
Beer	5%	39.5	545 ml	21.5
Wine	13%	103	175 ml / 250 ml	17.9/25.6

Figure 3.4. Concentrations of alcohol per serving.

TOXICITY

Adults absorb 80–90% of the alcohol they ingest within one hour and they metabolise it at a rate of 7–15 grams per hour. The fatal dose in adults is approximately 5–8 grams per kilogram body weight.

- A blood concentration of 1.8 g/l usually causes intoxication.
- A blood concentration of 3.5 g/l is associated with coma.
- A blood concentration of >4.5 g/l is often fatal.

FEATURES

- Mild alcohol toxicity leads to:
  - impaired visual acuity
  - impaired reaction time
  - impaired co-ordination
- Moderate alcohol toxicity leads to:
  - slurred speech
  - diplopia
  - blurred vision
  - ataxia
  - blackouts
  - sweating
  - loss of co-ordination
  - tachycardia
  - nausea and vomiting
  - hypoglycaemia – may be delayed for up to 36 hours
  - hypokalaemia
- Severe alcohol toxicity leads to:
  - hypothermia
  - hypotension
  - dilated pupils
  - depressed or absent tendon reflexes
  - coma
  - convulsions
  - respiratory depression
  - severe hypoglycaemia
  - metabolic acidosis
  - respiratory or cardiac arrest

ASSESSMENT AND INVESTIGATION OF ALCOHOL OVERDOSE

- Monitor blood pressure, pulse, temperature, respiratory rate and oxygen saturations.
- Monitor blood glucose.
- Obtain venous blood sample for U&E and blood alcohol levels.

- Obtain arterial blood gases.
- Obtain an ECG.
- Obtain a chest x-ray.

TREATMENT

- Use an ABC approach and commence CPR if required.
- Correct hypoglycaemia. If the patient is conscious give oral glucose.
- If the patient is unconscious, give 500 mls of 5% dextrose or 250 mls of 10% dextrose intravenously.
- Glucagon is not usually effective in this situation.
- If the patient is hypotensive, give 500 mls of gelofusine.
- If hypotension persists, inotropes may be required and medical assistance must be summoned immediately.
- Inotropes that may be used are:
  ➢ dopamine 2–10 micrograms/kg a minute
  ➢ dobutamine 2.5–10 micrograms/kg a minute.
- If hypothermic, re-warm at a rate of 1 °C per hour.
- Control convulsions with intravenous diazepam 0.1–0.3 mg /kg or lorazepam 4 mg.
- If fits are unresponsive, phenytoin at a loading dose of 15 mg/kg IV may help.
- If fits persist, urgent referral to ITU for intubation, sedation and ventilation may be necessary.
- If the blood alcohol concentration is >5 g/l, or if arterial pH <7.0, referral to the renal team for haemodialysis may be necessary.

THE NATIONAL INSTITUTE FOR CLINICAL EXCELLENCE (NICE) SELF-HARM GUIDELINE

The NICE self-harm clinical guideline was published in July 2004. The aim of this guideline is to provide healthcare professionals with a framework of consideration when dealing with patients who self-harm. It does not replace individual clinical judgement but healthcare professionals are expected to take this guidance into account when providing and planning care in conjunction with patients and their relatives. The full document can be found on the NICE website (see below). The key priorities of the guideline are as follows:

- People who have self-harmed should be treated with the same care, respect and privacy as any patient. In addition healthcare professionals should take account of the likely distress associated with self-harm.
- Clinical and non-clinical staff who have contact with people who self-harm in any setting should be provided with appropriate training to equip them to understand and care for people who have self-harmed.

- Ambulance and emergency department services whose staff may be involved in the care of people who have self-harmed by poisoning should ensure that activated charcoal is immediately available to staff at all times.
- All people who have self-harmed should be offered a preliminary psychosocial assessment at triage following an act of deliberate self-harm. Assessment should determine a person's mental capacity, their willingness to remain for further assessment, their level of distress and the possible presence of mental illness.
- Consideration should be given to introducing the Australian Mental Health Triage Scale, as it is a comprehensive assessment scale that provides an effective process for rating clinical urgency so that patients are seen in a timely manner.
- If a person who has self-harmed has to wait for treatment, he or she should be offered an environment that is safe and supportive and which minimises any distress. For many patients this may be a separate, quiet room with supervision and regular contact with a named member of staff to ensure safety.
- People who have self-harmed should be offered treatment for the physical consequences of self-harm, regardless of their willingness to accept psychosocial assessment or psychiatric treatment.
- Adequate analgesia/anaesthesia should be offered to people who have self-injured throughout the process of suturing or other painful treatments.
- Staff should provide full information about the treatment options and make all efforts necessary to ensure that someone who has self-harmed can give, and has the opportunity to give, meaningful and informed consent before any and each procedure or treatment is initiated.
- All people who have self-harmed should be offered an assessment of needs, which should be comprehensive and include evaluation of the social, psychological, and motivational factors specific to the act of self-harm, current suicidal intent, and hopelessness, as well as full mental health and social needs assessment.
- All people who have self-harmed should be assessed for risk. This assessment should include identification of the main clinical and demographic features known to be associated with risk of further self-harm and/or suicide and identification of the key psychological characteristics associated with the risk, in particular depression, hopelessness, and continuing suicidal intent.
- Following psychosocial assessment for people who have self-harmed, the decision about referral for further treatment and help should be based upon a comprehensive psychiatric, psychological, and social assessment, including an assessment of risk, and should not be determined solely on the basis of having self-harmed.

Source: National Institute for Clinical Excellence (2004): 'Key priorities for implementation'. In: Clinical Guideline 16: Self-harm: The short-term physical and psychological management and secondary prevention of self-harm in primary and secondary care. Quick Reference Guide. London: National Institute for Clinical Excellence. Available from www.nice.org.uk/CG016NICEguideline Reproduced with the permission of the National Institute for Health and Clinical Excellence.

ALCOHOL WITHDRAWAL

DEFINITION

Alcohol dependence is the physical and psychological dependence on alcohol. Any sudden cessation in the consumption in alcohol can lead to physical symptoms of withdrawal. These range from nausea and minor tremor to grand mal seizures (Kumar and Clark 2003). Alcohol dependence has seven essential elements. These are:

- a compulsive need to drink
- a regular drinking routine to avoid or relieve withdrawal symptoms
- drinking takes priority over other activities
- increased tolerance to alcohol
- repeated withdrawal symptoms often worse on waking in the morning
- early morning drinking to avoid withdrawal symptoms
- reinstatement after abstinence

SYMPTOMS AND SIGNS

Alcohol withdrawal can be classified as mild, moderate and severe. Mild withdrawal does not require hospital admission.

Mild Withdrawal

- mild anxiety
- some sweating
- a slight tremor
- insomnia
- tachycardia
- mild pyrexia
- hyper-reflexia
- nausea and vomiting
- diarrhoea

Moderate Withdrawal

- anxiety
- malaise
- depression
- irritability
- tremor
- pyrexia
- mild hypertension

Severe Withdrawal

- confusion
- anxiety
- insomnia
- sweating
- hallucinations
- disorientation
- restlessness
- coarse tremor
- ataxia
- tachycardia
- pyrexia
- hypertension
- vestibular disturbance
- convulsions

ASSESSMENT

Airway

- Ensure patent airway.
- Nurse in recovery position if unconscious.
- Utilise guedel airway or nasopharyngeal airway if necessary.
- Consider intubation if unable to maintain airway.

Breathing

- Give high-flow oxygen if unconscious.
- Monitor oxygen saturations.
- Monitor respiratory rate.
- Assist ventilation with bag valve mask if necessary.

Circulation

- Gain intravenous access.
- Record ECG.
- Monitor blood pressure.
- Obtain venous blood for FBC, U&E, LFTs, INR, calcium, magnesium and glucose.
- If the patient is suffering from moderate or severe withdrawal, obtain arterial blood gases.
- Record temperature.
- Give parenteral thiamine and ensure a further three doses are prescribed.

Disability

- Assess using AVPU or Glasgow Coma Scale.
- Take a detailed alcohol history if you have not already done so.
- Assess severity of withdrawal.
- Commence a withdrawal regime of diazepam or lorazepam.
- Use lorazepam if the patient has deranged LFTs or known liver disease.
- Use IV lorazepam if the patient is unable to swallow.
- If there is no evidence of liver disease, diazepam may be used.

The British Association of Pharmacology (2004) suggest the following as a reducing diazepam regime:

- Diazepam 10 mg QDS for 2 days followed by
- Diazepam 10 mg TDS for 2 days followed by
- Diazepam 5 mg QDS for 2 days followed by
- Diazepam 5 mg TDS for 2 days followed by
- Diazepam 5 mg BD for 2 days followed by
- Diazepam 5 mg OD for 2 days and stop.

Exposure

- Look for any injuries that may have been sustained during collapse or any seizure that may have occurred.
- The Driver and Vehicle Licensing Authority (DVLA) states that a person with alcohol dependence cannot drive a car until they have been abstinent for one year. It is therefore important to inform the patient if they hold a driving licence that they must inform the DVLA. Ensure this is documented in their medical notes.

DRUG WITHDRAWAL

DEFINITION

Drug dependence is the physical and psychological dependence on drugs such as opiates, cocaine, lysergide (LSD), benzodiazepines and amphetamines. Any sudden cessation in the consumption of these drugs can lead to physical symptoms of withdrawal.

The management of overdose of drugs has already been dealt with earlier in this chapter. Patients may present to MAU with the primary problem of drug withdrawal. This is not usually a medical emergency and requires referral to a specialist in addiction for management. However, some patients attending MAU may, as a result of admission with another medical problem, exhibit symptoms and signs of withdrawal from drugs as a secondary problem. It is therefore important that practitioners are able to recognise and manage this medical problem.

SYMPTOMS AND SIGNS

Patients withdrawing from drugs may present with varying symptoms depending on the drug they are addicted to. What follows is a list of typical symptoms and signs for the most common drugs abused:

Opiates

- sweating
- tachycardia
- leg cramps
- abdominal cramps
- nausea and vomiting
- diarrhoea
- dilated pupils
- sneezing
- running eyes and nose
- yawning
- piloerection
- withdrawal is often described as 'cold turkey'

Cocaine

- agitation
- tachycardia
- cardiac arrhythmias
- seizures
- pyrexia

LSD

- withdrawal is rare but can lead to a severe psychotic state

Benzodiazepines

- tremor
- agitation
- insomnia
- pyrexia
- weakness
- seizure
- confusion
- hyper-reflexia
- irritability
- nystagmus

Amphetamines

- confusion
- hallucinations
- cardiac arrhythmias
- violent behaviour can result from amphetamine use

ASSESSMENT

Airway

- Ensure patent airway.
- Nurse in recovery position if unconscious.
- Utilise guedel airway or nasopharyngeal airway if necessary.
- Consider intubation if unable to maintain airway.

Breathing

- Give high flow oxygen if unconscious.
- Monitor oxygen saturations – aim to maintain saturations >92%.
- Monitor respiratory rate.
- Assist ventilation with bag valve mask if necessary.

Circulation

- Gain intravenous access.
- Record ECG.
- Monitor blood pressure.
- Obtain venous blood for FBC, U&E, LFTs and glucose.
- Record temperature.

Disability

- Assess using AVPU or Glasgow Coma Scale.
- Take a detailed drug history if you have not already done so.
- Assess severity of withdrawal (Figure 3.5).
- Treat withdrawal symptomatically.
- If the patient requires an antiemetic and sedative, give promethiazine hydrochloride 25 mg orally every 12 hours.
- If the patient has somatic anxiety, give propanolol 40 mg orally every eight hours.
- For treatment of diarrhoea, give loperamide 4 mg orally as a single dose.
- For the treatment of stomach cramps, give hyoscine butylbromide 10–20 mg orally every eight hours.
- To relieve pain, give paracetamol 1 g orally every six hours or ibuprofen 400 mg orally every eight hours.
- For treatment of opiate withdrawal, obtain a witnessed urine sample.

For each item, circle the number that best describes the patient's signs or symptom. Rate on just the apparent relationship to opiate withdrawal. For example, if heart rate is increased because the patient was jogging just prior to assessment, the increased pulse rate would not add to the score.

Patient's Name:_____	Date and Time_____/_____/_____:_____
Reason for this	
assessment:____	

Resting Pulse Rate _____ beats/minute	**GI Upset** *over last $1/2$ hour*
measured after patient is sitting or lying for one minute	0 no GI symptoms
0 pulse rate 80 or below	1 stomach cramps
1 pulse rate 81–100	2 nausea or loose stool
2 pulse rate 101–120	3 vomiting or diarrhea
4 pulse rate greater than 120	5 Multiple episodes of diarrhea or vomiting
Sweating *over past $1/2$ hour not accounted for by room*	**Tremor** *observation of outstretched hands*
temperature or patient activity	0 no tremor
0 no report of chills or flushing	1 tremor can be felt, but not observed
1 subjective report of chills or flushing	2 slight tremor observable
2 flushed or observable moistness on face	4 gross tremor or muscle twitching
3 beads of sweat on brow or face	
4 sweat streaming off face	
Restlessness *observation during assessment*	**Yawning** *observation during assessment*
0 able to sit still	0 no yawning
1 reports difficulty sitting still, but is able to do so	1 yawning once or twice during assessment
3 frequent shifting or extraneous movements of legs/arms	2 yawning three or more times during assessment
5 unable to sit still for more than a few seconds	4 yawning several times/minute
Pupil Size	**Anxiety or Irritability**
0 pupils pinned or normal size for room light	0 none
1 pupils possibly larger than normal for room light	1 patient reports increasing irritability or anxiousness
2 pupils moderately dilated	2 patient obviously irritable or anxious
5 pupils so dilated that only the rim of the iris is visible	4 patient so irritable or anxious that participation in the assessment is difficult
Bone or Joint Aches *if patient was having pain*	**Gooseflesh Skin**
previously, only the additional component attributed	0 skin is smooth
to opiates withdrawal is scored	3 piloerection of skin can be felt or hairs standing up
0 not present	on arms
1 mild diffuse discomfort	5 prominent piloerection
2 patient reports severe diffuse aching of joints / muscles	
4 patient is rubbing joints or muscles and is unable to sit still because of discomfort	
Runny Nose or Tearing *not accounted for by cold*	
symptoms or allergies	Total score _____
0 not present	The total score is the sum of all 11 items
1 nasal stuffiness or unusually moist eyes	Initials of person
2 nose running or tearing	completing Assessment:
4 nose constantly running or tears streaming down cheeks	

Score: 5–12 = mild; 13–24 = moderate; 25–36 = moderately severe; more than 36 = severe withdrawal

Figure 3.5. Clinical opiate withdrawal scale.

- If witnessed urine confirms use of opiates, a substitution regime with methadone can be commenced. This may vary according to local policy, so check local policies before treatment is commenced.
- A scoring system as in Figure 3.5 is utilised to assess severity of withdrawal and methadone prescribed in accordance with severity.

Exposure

- If you have not already done so, obtain a witnessed urine sample for narcotic assessment.
- Look for any injuries that may have been sustained.
- The DVLA states that anyone with an addiction to heroin, cocaine or benzodi-azepines cannot drive a car until they have been free from the use of these drugs for one year, after which their licence may be reinstated providing the DVLA is in receipt of an independent negative urine screen. It is therefore important that you tell the patient they must inform the DVLA and document this in the medical notes.
- If a patient is on a consultant supervised oral methadone programme, they may hold a driving licence which is subject to annual review.

REFERENCES

Bailey B and McGuigan MA (1998) Management of anaphylactoid reactions to intravenous N-acetylcysteine. *Annals of Emergency Medicine* 31: 710–15.

British Association of Pharmacology (2004) Evidence based guideline for the pharmacological management of substance misuse, addiction and co-morbidity. *Journal of Psychopharmacology* 18(3): 293–335.

Department of Health (2005) *Nurse Prescribers Extended Formulary*. London: DoH.

Flanagan RJ and Meredith TJ (1991) Use of N-acetylcysteine in clinical toxicology. *American Journal of Medicine* 91: Suppl 3c.

Johnson RA (1982) Survival after a serum ethanol concentration of 1.5%. *Lancet* 1394.

Krause DS, Wolf BA and Shaw LM (1992) Acute aspirin overdose: mechanisms of toxicity. *Therapeutic Drug Monitoring* 14: 441–51.

National Institute for Clinical Excellence (2004) *Self Harm. Clinical Guideline* 16. Key priorities for implementation, pp. 5–6. London: NICE.

Office for National Statistics (2005) *Deaths by Misuse of Drugs in England 2003–2004*. London: Office for National Statistics.

Resuscitation Council (UK) (2005) *Resuscitation Guidelines 2005*, ed. A Handley. London: Resuscitation Council.

Royal College of Physicians (2001) *Alcohol: Can the NHS Afford It?* London: Royal College of Physicians.

Teasdale G and Jennett B (1974) The Glasgow Coma Scale. *Lancet* (ii) 81–3.

Toxbase, accessed via www.spib.axl.co.uk

Watson WA (1998) Opioid toxicity recurrence after an initial response to naloxone. *Clinical Toxicology* 36: 11–17.

4 Infection

SEPSIS AND SEPTIC SHOCK

Sepsis and septic shock are life-threatening. Overall mortality ranges from 25% to 90%. Poor results often follow failure to institute therapy soon enough. It is therefore vital that as a nurse practitioner you can recognise the septic patient, initiate treatment, and obtain prompt assistance (Dellinger et al. 2004).

DEFINITION

Sepsis is a systemic response to bacteraemia. When bacteraemia produces changes in circulation such that tissue perfusion is critically reduced, septic shock ensues (Dellinger et al. 2004).

Approximately 40% of patients with sepsis are as a result of gram-positive organisms and 60% as a result of gram-negative organisms. Fungi are less common but should never be discounted (Kumar and Clark 2003).

In previously healthy adults consider the chest, urinary tract or biliary tree as the most common sources of infection. In a hospitalised patient the source may be a wound, an indwelling urinary catheter or intravenous catheter.

In a patient who is known to abuse intravenous drugs septicaemia may be caused by different organisms. The most likely organisms are staphylococcus aureus and pseudomonas sp.

SYMPTOMS AND SIGNS

Patients with sepsis and septic shock are acutely ill. Prompt assessment and treatment is vital. Patients can and do die from sepsis. For this reason medical assistance will be required. Summon help immediately. Common symptoms are:

- rigors and fever
- sweating
- headache
- muscle pain

Look for a source of primary infection. Some have been mentioned previously but consider the following:

- urinary tract infection
- respiratory tract infection

- skin infections
- meningitis (to be covered later in this chapter)
- infective endocarditis (to be covered later in this chapter)
- intra abdominal infection
- osteomyelitis
- pelvic inflammatory disease
- sexually transmitted disease

Patients with sepsis present with:

- circulatory disturbance
- poor peripheral perfusion
- tachycardia
- tachypnoea
- pyrexia or temperature $<36\,°C$
- hypotension

ASSESSMENT

As always, utilise an ABCDE approach to assessment.

Airway

- Ensure airway is patent (head tilt chin left if necessary).
- Utilise airway adjuncts if necessary (guedel or nasopharyngeal airway).
- If airway is compromised contact anaesthetist and ICU immediately for possible rapid sequence induction (RSI).

Breathing

- Assess respiratory rate – >24 breaths/min is significant.
- Assess oxygen saturations.
- Obtain arterial blood gases – to assess oxygenation and the presence of acidosis.
- Give 100% oxygen via non re-breath mask.
- Auscultate chest – are there signs of a chest infection?
- Request chest x-ray.

Circulation

- Assess heart rate – >100 beats/min is significant.
- Monitor blood pressure – systolic BP <90 mmHg is poor prognostic sign.
- Check capillary refill time.
- Gain intravenous access via two large bore cannulae.
- Give colloid via IV access – gelofusin or haemaccel.
- Insert urinary catheter.

- Obtain venous blood for FBC, U&E, LFTs, CRP and INR.
- Obtain blood cultures.
- Obtain samples of urine and sputum for culture and sensitivity.
- Record temperature – the patient may have pyrexia or temperature may be <36 °C.
- Commence broad spectrum antibiotics intravenously – this will depend on individual local antibiotic policies. Cefuroxime, Tazocin or Gentamicin are typical examples.

Disability

Confusion is often one of the first signs of sepsis in the previously fit and well adult.

- Assess level of consciousness using AVPU score.

Exposure

If the source of infection is not known, look for injury, wounds, injection sites and any other source of infection.

LIFE-THREATENING FEATURES

Severe sepsis is defined as sepsis in the presence of impaired organ function.
   If any of the following life threatening features are present urgent referral to ICU is indicated.

- diminished renal function
- impaired cardiac function
- hypoxia
- acidosis
- clotting disturbance
- acute respiratory distress syndrome (ARDS) – cardinal feature is pulomonary oedema; the patient has stiff lungs, refractory hypoaxaemia and bilateral pulmonary infiltrates on CXR

Septic shock is defined as severe sepsis with a systolic blood pressure of <90 mmHg

MENINGITIS

Suspected meningitis is a fairly common referral to the medical assessment unit. This is probably due to the degree of government and media publicity dedicated to raising awareness of the signs and symptoms of meningitis. Thankfully the majority of these admissions for suspected meningitis are proved not to be meningitis. The overall mortality rate is 10% (British Infection Society supported by the Meningitis Research Foundation 2003). Therefore prompt recognition and assessment is required.

DEFINITION

Meningitis is inflammation of the pia and arachnoid mater or meninges, which are membranous tissues that surround the brain. The term meningitis is usually reserved for inflammation as a result of infection. There are three common presentations:

• meningitis alone
• septicaemia alone
• meningococcal septicaemia – an overlap of the two

Meningitis is characterised by the presence of:

• fever
• headache
• neck stiffness
• photophobia and vomiting
• confusion (may be present)

Septicaemic patients frequently do not show signs of neurological impairment. As discussed previously in this chapter septicaemic patients present with:

• circulatory disturbance
• poor peripheral perfusion
• tachycardia
• tachypnoea
• hypotension
• presence of a petichial rash indicates that the patient is bacteraemic with meningo-cocci

ASSESSMENT

As always, utilise an ABCDE approach to assessment.

Airway

• Ensure airway is patent (head tilt chin left if necessary).
• Utilise airway adjuncts if necessary (guedel or nasopharyngeal airway).
• If airway is compromised contact anaesthetist and ICU immediately for possible rapid sequence induction (RSI).

Breathing

• Assess respiratory rate – <8 or >30 is significant.
• Assess oxygen saturations.
• Obtain arterial blood gases.
• Give 100% oxygen via non re-breath mask.
• Auscultate chest.
• Request chest x-ray.

Circulation

- Assess heart rate – >100 or <40 beats/min is significant.
- Monitor blood pressure – systolic BP <90 mmHg is poor prognostic sign.
- Check capillary refill time.
- Gain intravenous access via two large bore cannulae.
- Give colloid via IV access – gelofusin or haemaccel.
- Insert urinary catheter.
- Obtain venous blood for FBC, U&E, LFTs, CRP and INR.
- Obtain EDTA blood for meningitis PCR.
- Obtain blood cultures.
- Obtain throat swab for culture and sensitivity.
- Record temperature – may have pyrexia or temperature may be <36 °C.

Disability

- Assess level of consciousness using AVPU score.
- Observe for focal neurological signs – persistent seizures, papilloedema.

Exposure

- Observe for signs of petechial rash.

LIFE-THREATENING FEATURES

If the patient demonstrates any of the following signs urgent medical assistance is required and the patient needs review by ICU.

- rapidly progressive rash
- CRT >4 seconds
- oliguria
- respiratory rate <8 or >30 breaths/min
- heart rate <40 or >140 beats/min
- acidosis pH <7.3 or BE worse than −5
- WBC <4
- marked depressed conscious level – GCS <12 or a fall in GCS of >2
- focal neurology
- persistent seizures
- bradycardia and hypertension
- papilloedema

The Meningitis Research Foundation in conjunction with the British Infection Society has developed an algorithm for the early management of suspected bacterial meningitis and this should be used as a guide to investigation and treatment.

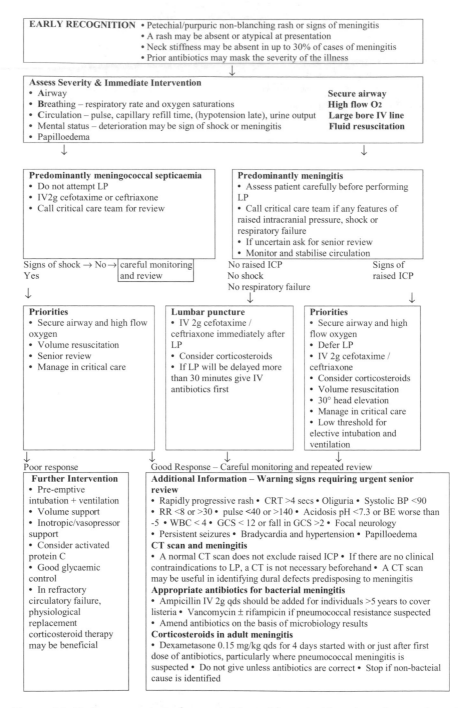

EARLY RECOGNITION • Petechial/purpuric non-blanching rash or signs of meningitis
• A rash may be absent or atypical at presentation
• Neck stiffness may be absent in up to 30% of cases of meningitis
• Prior antibiotics may mask the severity of the illness

↓

Assess Severity & Immediate Intervention
• Airway   **Secure airway**
• Breathing – respiratory rate and oxygen saturations   **High flow O₂**
• Circulation – pulse, capillary refill time, (hypotension late), urine output   **Large bore IV line**
• Mental status – deterioration may be sign of shock or meningitis   **Fluid resuscitation**
• Papilloedema

↓   ↓

Predominantly meningococcal septicaemia
• Do not attempt LP
• IV2g cefotaxime or ceftriaxone
• Call critical care team for review

Predominantly meningitis
• Assess patient carefully before performing LP
• Call critical care team if any features of raised intracranial pressure, shock or respiratory failure
• If uncertain ask for senior review
• Monitor and stabilise circulation

Signs of shock → No → | careful monitoring and review | No raised ICP   Signs of
Yes   No shock   raised ICP
                                                           No respiratory failure
↓   ↓   ↓

Priorities
• Secure airway and high flow oxygen
• Volume resuscitation
• Senior review
• Manage in critical care

Lumbar puncture
• IV 2g cefotaxime / ceftriaxone immediately after LP
• Consider corticosteroids
• If LP will be delayed more than 30 minutes give IV antibiotics first

Priorities
• Secure airway and high flow oxygen
• Defer LP
• IV 2g cefotaxime / ceftriaxone
• Consider corticosteroids
• Volume resuscitation
• 30° head elevation
• Manage in critical care
• Low threshold for elective intubation and ventilation

↓   ↓   ↓
Poor response   Good Response – Careful monitoring and repeated review

Further Intervention
• Pre-emptive intubation + ventilation
• Volume support
• Inotropic/vasopressor support
• Consider activated protein C
• Good glycaemic control
• In refractory circulatory failure, physiological replacement corticosteroid therapy may be beneficial

Additional Information – Warning signs requiring urgent senior review
• Rapidly progressive rash • CRT >4 secs • Oliguria • Systolic BP <90 • RR <8 or >30 • pulse <40 or >140 • Acidosis pH <7.3 or BE worse than -5 • WBC < 4 • GCS < 12 or fall in GCS >2 • Focal neurology • Persistent seizures • Bradycardia and hypertension • Papilloedema
CT scan and meningitis
• A normal CT scan does not exclude raised ICP • If there are no clinical contraindications to LP, a CT is not necessary beforehand • A CT scan may be useful in identifying dural defects predisposing to meningitis
Appropriate antibiotics for bacterial meningitis
• Ampicillin IV 2g qds should be added for individuals >5 years to cover listeria • Vancomycin ± rifampicin if pneumococcal resistance suspected • Amend antibiotics on the basis of microbiology results
Corticosteroids in adult meningitis
• Dexametasone 0.15 mg/kg qds for 4 days started with or just after first dose of antibiotics, particularly where pneumococcal meningitis is suspected • Do not give unless antibiotics are correct • Stop if non-bacteial cause is identified

Figure 4.1. Early management of suspected bacterial meningitis and menigococcal septi-caemia in immunocompetent adults. Reproduced with kind permission of Heyderman et al. (2003) Early management of suspected bacterial meningitis and menigococcal septicaemia in immunocompetent adults. *Journal of Infection* 46(2): 75–7.

FURTHER INVESTIGATION AND MANAGEMENT

If you have managed the patient on your own up until this point, now is the time to call for expert medical help.

- A lumbar puncture (LP) should be considered.
- A CT scan is not always necessary prior to LP. A normal CT scan does not exclude raised intracranial pressure. If there are no clinical contraindications to lumbar puncture, a CT scan is not necessary beforehand.
- If the patient has predominantly meningococcal septicaemia, following assessment an LP is not indicated.
- If the patient has predominantly meningitis, consider an LP.
- In either case give 2g IV cefotaxime or ceftriaxone – if LP performed do not give until after LP.
- Antibiotics may need to be amended following microbiology results.
- If you are confident that you are using the correct antimicrobials, consider Dexametasone 0.15 mg/kg qds for four days (De Gan and Van de Beek 2002).
- If probable or confirmed meningococcal disease inform Public Health and assist with contact tracing as contacts will need prophylaxis treatment.

INFECTIVE ENDOCARDITIS

Infective endocarditis (IE) carries a high risk of morbidity and mortality (Bayer et al. 1998). Rapid diagnosis, effective treatment and prompt recognition of complications are essential to good patient outcome. The input of specialists to aid diagnosis and treatment will be required.

DEFINITION

Infective endocarditis is an infection of the endocardium or vascular endothelium of the heart. The presentation of infective endocarditis is highly variable and may affect almost any organ. The symptoms may be non-specific and of insidious onset.

Infection occurs in the following cases:

- On valves which have a congenital or acquired defect – usually on the left side of the heart.
- Right-sided endocarditis is more common in intravenous drug users.
- On normal valves.
- On prosthetic valves.
- In association with ventricular septal defect, persitent ductus arteriosus and coarctation of the aorta.

Other risk factors include:

- previous IE
- known aortic or mitral regurgitation

- aortic stenosis
- intravenous drug abuse
- immunosuppressed patients
- patients with an indwelling intravenous catheter
- rheumatic heart disease

The most common organisms causing endocarditis are:

- Streptococcus mutans and sanguis – these organisms are present in the upper respiratory tract. Bacteraemia occurs after dental extraction, tonsillectomy and bronchoscopy.
- Enterococcus faecalis – particularly common following invasive genitourinary or gastrointestinal investigation or procedure.
- Staphylococcus aureus – particularly common in intravenous drug users, patients with central venous lines and patients with prosthetic valves.
- Streptococcus bovis, candida albicans, coxiella burnetii and chlamydia psittaci are more uncommon causative organisms.

SYMPTOMS AND SIGNS

Patients usually present with systemic features of infection. Common features are:

- malaise
- fever
- night sweats
- anorexia and weight loss
- nausea and vomiting
- shortness of breath
- musculoskeletal pain

ASSESSMENT

As always, utilise an ABCDE approach to assessment.

Airway

- Ensure airway is patent (head tilt chin left if necessary).
- Utilise airway adjuncts if necessary (guedel or nasopharyngeal airway).
- If airway is compromised contact anaesthetist and ICU immediately for possible rapid sequence induction (RSI).

Breathing

- Assess respiratory rate.
- Assess oxygen saturations.

- Obtain arterial blood gases if patient is hypoxic on pulse oximetry.
- Give 100% oxygen via non re-breath mask if patient is hypoxic.
- Auscultate chest – listen for signs of oedema.
- Request chest x-ray – for signs of heart failure.

Circulation

- Assess heart rate and listen for heart sounds – a new mitral, aortic or tricuspid murmur is highly suggestive of endocarditis.
- Observe for signs of clubbing – usually present in prolonged disease.
- Monitor blood pressure.
- Gain intravenous access.
- Obtain venous blood for FBC and differential white count, U&E, LFTs, CRP, ESR, INR and complement, C3, C4 and CH50.
- Obtain blood cultures – three sets from three separate sites over a 24-hour period.
- Obtain sample of urine for protein and microscopic haematuria.
- Record temperature.
- Obtain ECG to look for conduction abnormality.
- An echo is required to identify vegetations and underlying valvular dysfunction – transoesophageal echo is a more sensitive test and referral to a cardiologist should be made urgently.

Disability

- Assess level of consciousness using AVPU score.

Exposure

Further physical examination should be undertaken once the patient is stable to identify other clinical signs indicative of endocarditis. Indicative signs are:

- mucuocutaneous petechiae
- Janeway lesions – painless haemorrhagic, macular plaques most commonly seen on the palms and soles of the feet
- Roth spots – small retinal haemorrhages with pale centres seen near the optic nerve on fundoscopy
- splinter haemorrhages – seen under nail beds
- signs of anaemia
- signs of splenomegaly – perform abdominal examination

Durack et al. (1994) developed the Duke Clinical Criteria for diagnosis of IE. This should be utilised when dealing with a patient with suspected IE.

Classification	Criteria
Definite clinical IE	Two major clinical criteria (see Figure 4.3) **or** one major and three minor criteria **or** five minor criteria
Probable IE	Clinical findings consistent with IE but fall short of 'definite' and cannot be 'rejected'
Reject diagnosis	Firm alternative diagnosis for manifestations of IE and resolution of manifestations without antibiotic therapy or with antibiotic therapy of ≤ four days

Figure 4.2. Duke classification in the diagnosis of IE. Reproduced with kind permission of Elsevier.

Criteria	Definition
Major criteria	**1. Positive blood culture for IE** A. Typical micro-organisms from 2 separate blood cultures i) *Strep viridans, Strep. Bovis, Haemophilus spp., Cardiobacterium hominis, Eikenella spp., or Kingella spp.* **or** ii) Community acquired *Staph aureus or enterococci* in the absence of a primary focus B. Blood culture persistently positive for organisms consistent with IE i) Two positive cultures drawn >12 hours apart **or** ii) all of three, or majority of ≥4 cultures (where first and last sample drawn >1 hour apart) **2. Evidence of endocardial involvement** A. Positive echocardiogram for IE i) oscillating intracardiac mass on valve or supporting structures **or** ii) abcess **or** iii) new partial dehiscence of prosthetic valve B. New valvular regurgitation **3. Positive serology for causes of culture negative IE** i) Q-fever (Coxiella burnetti) **or** ii) e.g. Bartonella, Chlamydia psittaci **4. Identification of micro-organism from blood or tissue using molecular biology**
Minor criteria	1. Predisposition: predisposing heart condition or IV drug use 2. Fever: temperature >38°C 3. Vascular phenomenon: major arterial emboli, septic pulmonary infarct, mycotic aneurysm, intracranial haemorrhage, conjunctival haemorrhage, Janeway lesions, newly diagnosed clubbing, splinter haemorrhages, splenomegaly 4. Immunogenic phenomena: glomerulonephritis, Roth spots, RhF +ve, high ESR, CRP >100 mg/l 5. Microbiogical evidence: positive blood cultures not meeting definition of major criteria or serological evidence of active organism consistent with IE 6. Echocardiographic evidence of IE which does not meet major criteria

Figure 4.3. Definitions of Duke clinical criteria. Reproduced with kind permission of Elsevier.

TREATMENT

- In patients who are stable do not start antibiotics until at least three separate sets of blood cultures have been taken.
- In an ill patient do not wait for blood culture results or an echo before starting antibiotic treatment.
- Treatment is with intravenous antibiotics for a minimum of two weeks followed by a further course of oral antibiotics for 2–4 weeks.
- while awaiting blood culture results IV benzylpenicillin 1.2 g four-hourly and gentamicin 80 mg IV 12 hourly should be given.
- If the patient is allergic to penicillin, vancomycin 1g IV 12 hourly by slow intravenous infusion should be given in conjunction with gentamicin.
- Subsequent treatment will depend on the culture sensitivities.

COMPLICATIONS AND SURGICAL INTERVENTION

Be aware that complications can arise and prompt referral to expert medical help must be made if any of the following occur:

- heart failure
- vegetation embolisation – emboli threaten a limb or an organ with potential organ failure or loss of a limb
- metastatic abcess – pneumonia or lung abcess; this is a particular risk in right-sided endocarditis
- abcess in aortic valve ring – can lead to complete heart block
- immune complex disease – symptoms of a vasculitic rash, arthiritis, glomerulonephritis

Early surgical intervention and therefore urgent referral to the cardiothoracic surgeons is indicated in the following:

- heart failure
- progressive valve damage
- a conduction defect
- recurrent embolism
- resistant infection – especially associated with prosthetic valve
- fungal endocarditis

GASTROENTERITIS

DEFINITION

Gastroenteritis is diarrhoea with or without vomiting caused by the ingestion of bacteria, viruses or toxins. Often the cause is not found. However, contaminated food and water are the most frequent sources of infection. Some of the more common organisms are:

- staphylococcus aureus – from contaminated food and water – incubation 2–4 hours
- E coli 0157:H7 – from meat and milk – incubation 12–48 hours
- campylobacter jejuni – from meat and milk – incubation 48–96 hours
- salmonella spp – from meat and eggs – incubation 12–48 hours
- rotavirus – may be food or water borne – incubation 1–7 days

SYMPTOMS AND SIGNS

The common features of gastroenteritis are:

- diarrhoea
- vomiting
- nausea
- abdominal cramps
- malaise
- fever

ASSESSMENT

As always, utilise an ABCDE approach to assessment.

Airway

- Ensure airway is patent (head tilt chin left if necessary).
- Utilise airway adjuncts if necessary (guedel or nasopharyngeal airway).
- If airway is compromised, contact anaesthetist and ICU immediately for possible rapid sequence induction (RSI).

Breathing

- Assess respiratory rate.
- Assess oxygen saturations.
- Give oxygen if hypoxia is present – maintain saturations >92%.
- Auscultate chest.
- Request erect chest x-ray if perforation suspected.

Circulation

- Assess heart rate.
- Monitor blood pressure.
- Check capillary refill time.
- Gain intravenous access.

- Give IV fluids if patient dehydrated.
- Obtain venous blood for FBC, U&E, LFTs, CRP and INR.
- Record temperature.
- Obtain blood cultures if pyrexial.
- Maintain a strict fluid balance chart.
- Encourage oral fluids.
- If nausea and vomiting persist, prescribe an antiemetic IV.

Disability

- Assess level of consciousness using AVPU score.

Exposure

- Undertake a detailed history.
- Obtain information on the food and drink consumed recently.
- Obtain information on the time until onset of symptoms.
- Ascertain if other family members/friends are affected.
- Has there been any foreign travel?
- Undertake an abdominal examination.
- Request an abdominal x-ray.
- Obtain stool samples for microscopy, culture and sensitivity.
- Do not prescribe an antidiarrhoeal such as codeine or loperamide until stool culture results are known.
- Antibiotics should be withheld until stool culture results are known unless the patient is systemically very unwell, in which case they can be considered in conjunction with advice from microbiology.
- Remember – food poisoning is a notifiable disease in the UK – ensure the consultant in Communicable Disease Control is informed.

URINARY TRACT INFECTION (UTI)

DEFINITION

A UTI is defined as infection of any part of the urinary tract with bacteria. It is most commonly caused by the patient's own bowel flora but can also be caused by skin organisms. UTIs are more common in women than men. Worldwide 20% of women will suffer from a UTI at some stage in their life. UTIs are classified as uncomplicated or complicated.

Uncomplicated UTI – infection in a patient with no underlying renal or neurological disease.

Complicated UTI – infection in men or in the presence of underlying structural, renal or neurological disease.

Common organisms are:

- E coli
- staphylococcus saprophyticus
- enterococcus faecalis
- klebsiella species
- proteus mirabilis
- enterobacter species

SYMPTOMS AND SIGNS

Patients commonly present with the following:

- dysuria
- urgency
- frequency
- a feeling of bladder fullness
- haematuria
- offensive (smelly) urine
- suprapubic pain

Left untreated and in severe cases a UTI can migrate along the renal tract and the patient may develop acute pyelonephritis. Progression to pyelonephritis is associated with substantial morbidity. Patients can develop urethral obstruction, septic shock and perinephric abcess. Chronic pyelonephritis may lead to scarring and diminished renal function.

SYMPTOMS AND SIGNS OF PYELONEPHRITIS

- fever
- vomiting
- hypotension
- dehydration
- malaise
- loin pain
- renal angle tenderness

ASSESSMENT

As always, utilise an ABCDE approach to assessment.

Airway

- Ensure airway is patent (head tilt chin left if necessary).
- Utilise airway adjuncts if necessary (guedel or nasopharyngeal airway).
- If airway is compromised, contact anaesthetist and ICU immediately for possible rapid sequence induction (RSI).

Breathing

- Assess respiratory rate.
- Assess oxygen saturations.
- Give high-flow oxygen if saturations <92% and patient demonstrating signs of shock.
- Auscultate chest.
- Request chest x-ray if patient is shocked; otherwise it may not be necessary at this stage.

Circulation

- Assess heart rate.
- Monitor blood pressure.
- Check capillary refill time.
- Gain intravenous access.
- Give IV fluids if patient dehydrated or signs of shock are present.
- Obtain venous blood for FBC, U&E and CRP.
- Record temperature.
- Obtain blood cultures if pyrexial.
- Maintain a strict fluid balance chart.
- Encourage oral fluids.
- If nausea and vomiting present, prescribe an antiemetic IV.
- Undertake an abdominal examination.
- Obtain a urine dipstick and send a mid-stream urine (MSU) for microscopy, culture and sensitivity.
- Commence antibiotics if urine dipstick is positive – don't forget these may need to be altered once sensitivities are known.
- If urine dipstick is negative, wait for the results of the MSU before starting antibiotic therapy.

Disability

- Assess level of consciousness using AVPU score.

Exposure

- Undertake a detailed history if not already done so.
- Consider referral for an ultrasound scan of kidneys and urinary bladder if symptoms are recurrent or there are signs of pyelonephritis.

FEVER IN THE RETURNING TRAVELLER

DEFINITION

This is defined as a pyrexia in any person who has recently travelled to a foreign country (usually outside of Europe). Recent travel would normally be defined as within the last three months; however, certain illnesses such as hepatitis, tuberculosis (TB), malaria and amoebic liver abcess can take longer than this to manifest themselves, so this should be taken into consideration in anyone with a history of foreign travel in the last six months.

Some of the more common conditions that should be considered in the returning traveller are:

- falciparum malaria – the most common cause of fever in travellers to the tropics
- viral hepatitis
- dengue fever
- typhoid and paratyphoid
- gastroenteritis
- TB
- rickettsia
- amoebic liver abcess
- acute HIV infection
- febrile illness unrelated to foreign travel

In approximately a quarter of all cases of fever in the foreign traveller no obvious cause will be found, the illness will be self-limiting and they will be discharged home. However some illnesses if left untreated can be rapidly fatal and therefore prompt assessment and investigation are vital.

SYMPTOMS AND SIGNS

Patients may complain of non-specific symptoms. However, the most common complaints are:

- fever
- myalgia
- headache
- sore throat
- cough
- sputum production
- change in bowel habit – usually diarrhoea
- frequency of micturition
- dysuria
- nocturia
- soft tissue infection
- jaundice
- rash
- photophobia

Some of the disease specific complaints are:

- splenomegaly – acute/chronic malaria, schistosomiasis, visceral leishmaniosis
- hepatomegaly and jaundice – viral hepatitis
  ➤ with intercostal point tenderness – amoebic liver abcess

- altered mental state – cerebral malaria and typhoid
- myalgia, arthalgia and retro-orbital headache, rash and bleeding gums – dengue fever
- headache, myalgia, macular rash and lymphadenopathy – rickettsia
- hepatorenal failure with DIC – leptospirosis leading to Weil's disease
- headache, myalgia, cough and urticaria – schistosomiasis

ADVERSE FEATURES

- heart rate >120 bpm
- WCC >15
- temperature >39°C
- BP <90/60 mmHg
- postural BP drop
- cold peripheries
- rash
- drowsiness or altered GCS
- hypoxia
- acidosis
- respiratory distress
- diarrhoea
- vomiting
- inability to stand
- CRP >100
- DIC

ASSESSMENT

As always, utilise an ABCDE approach to assessment.

Airway

- Ensure airway is patent (head tilt chin left if necessary).
- Utilise airway adjuncts if necessary (guedel or nasopharyngeal airway).
- If airway is compromised, contact anaesthetist and ICU immediately for possible rapid sequence induction (RSI).

Breathing

- Assess respiratory rate.
- Assess oxygen saturations.
- Give high-flow oxygen if saturations <92% and patient demonstrating signs of shock.
- Auscultate chest.
- Request chest x-ray.

Circulation

- Assess heart rate.
- Monitor blood pressure.
- Check capillary refill time.
- Gain intravenous access.
- Give IV fluids if patient dehydrated or hypotensive.
- Obtain venous blood for FBC and differential, U&E and CRP.
- Discuss with microbiology the need for PCR.
- Record temperature.
- Obtain blood cultures.
- Obtain thick and thin film – this will need to continue after admission for three consecutive days.
- Obtain a throat swab.
- Obtain sputum for MC&S.
- Obtain stool for MC&S.
- Consider the need for a lumbar puncture in order to obtain CSF for culture and sensitivity.
- Maintain a strict fluid balance chart.
- Encourage oral fluids.
- Obtain a urine dipstick and send a mid-stream urine (MSU) for microscopy, culture and sensitivity.
- Withhold antibiotics until results of cultures are known.
- If the patient is severely ill, a broad spectrum antibiotic can be commenced – discuss with microbiology as to which is best.

Disability

- Assess level of consciousness using AVPU score.
- This should be repeated at regular intervals.
- Monitor blood sugar.

Exposure

Undertake a detailed history if not already done so – this should include:

- The onset, duration and exact nature of symptoms.
- Travel history:
  - places visited
  - mode of travel
  - exposure to potential hazards.
- Time spent in rural areas.
- Contact with fresh water.
- Sexual contacts.
- Food consumed.

- Immunisation history.
- Malaria prophylaxis compliance.
- Date of return to the UK.

All patients who have returned from foreign travel and have a pyrexia should be nursed in a side room, ideally with negative pressure. Once the nature of the illness is known the need for this can be reviewed.

NOTIFIABLE DISEASES

Certain diseases are notifiable to the consultant in Communicable Diseases. These are:

- diptheria
- amoebic and bacillary dysentery
- acute encephalitis
- food poisoning
- leptospirosis
- malaria
- meningitis
- meningococcal septicaemia
- scarlet fever
- typhoid and paratyphoid
- TB
- viral hepatitis
- viral haemorrhagic fever
- yellow fever
- whooping cough

HOT SWOLLEN JOINTS

DEFINITION

Any patient presenting with a hot swollen joint should be treated as if they have septic arthritis until it is proven otherwise.

Septic or pyogenic arthritis is defined as an infection producing inflammation in a native or prosthetic joint. It can be acute or chronic. In the acute form the most common infecting organism is staph. aureus. In chronic disease a wider range of organisms are involved.

This section will concentrate on the management of the acute, hot swollen joint.

Hot swollen joints occur in approximately 7 per every 100,000 head of population. They are most common in children and the elderly, especially males. Approximately 0.2–2% of all joint replacements are complicated by infection.

SYMPTOMS AND SIGNS

Patients with hot swollen joints present in the following cases:

- a short history of a hot, swollen and tender joint
- there is usually restriction of movement
- fever may be present
- erythema may be present
- vomiting
- hypotension

If vomiting and hypotension are present, treat the patient as having sepsis and follow the management of sepsis section at the beginning of this chapter.

The most commonly affected joints are:

- knee
- elbow
- hip
- wrist
- ankle

ASSESSMENT

In July 2006 the British Society of Rheumatology (BSR) issued guidance on the management of hot swollen joints in adults. This guidance is reflected in this section and the algorithm for management can be seen in Figure 4.4.

As always, utilise an ABCDE approach to assessment.

Airway

- Ensure airway is patent.
- Utilise airway adjuncts if necessary.
- If airway is compromised, contact anaesthetist and ICU immediately.

Breathing

- Assess respiratory rate.
- Assess oxygen saturations.
- Give oxygen via non re-breath mask to maintain saturations >92%.
- Auscultate chest.
- Request chest x-ray if appropriate.

Circulation

- Assess heart rate.
- Monitor blood pressure.

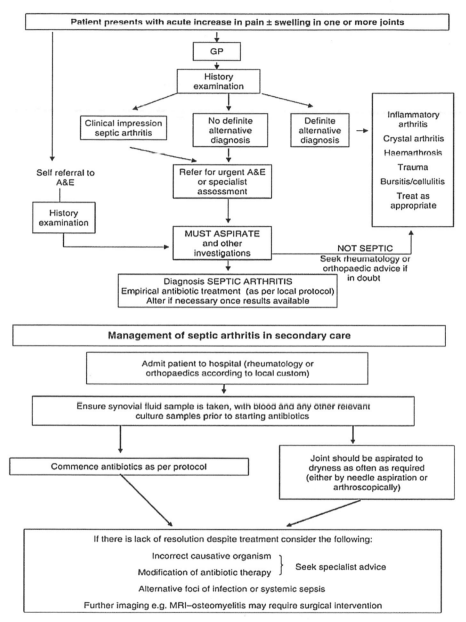

Figure 4.4. Algorithm for Management of Hot Swollen Joints. Reproduced with kind permission of the BSR and Oxford University Press.

- Gain intravenous access.
- Obtain venous blood sample for FBC, U&E, LFTs, ESR and CRP.
- If signs of sepsis are present:
  - ➤ summon help
  - ➤ follow sepsis management at the beginning of this chapter.
- Obtain blood cultures.
- Record temperature.
- Do not commence antibiotic therapy until synovial fluid has been aspirated.
- If you have not already done so, refer patient to orthopaedics or rheumatology depending on local policy as they require synovial fluid aspiration.

Disability

- Assess level of consciousness using AVPU.
- Exam the affected joint and all other joints for signs of inflammation.
- Obtain plain x-ray of the affected joint.
- Record BM.

Exposure

- If you have not already done so obtain a detailed history.
- Examine all other joints for signs of swelling and tenderness.
- Ensure that expert help is on its way to undertake synovial fluid aspiration. This should be Gram-stained and cultured.
- Once aspiration has been performed antibiotic therapy can be commenced.

ANTIBIOTIC THERAPY

Antibiotics should be commenced in accordance with local policy. However, the BSR has issued some guidance for the suggested antibiotic regimen.

ANTIMICROBIAL RESISTANCE

Antimicrobial resistance is the ability of micro-organisms to resist the growth-suppressing or microcidal effects of particular antimicrobial agents.

In 1998 the Department of Health released a document entitled *The Path of Least Resistance*. This highlighted the problems faced by antimicrobial resistance. Health-care professionals have a duty to reduce this worrying problem. By following some simple rules we can reduce antimicrobial resistance.

- Know your local microbiology and antibiotic policies.
- Before prescribing any antibiotic ask yourself, 'Does this patient really need an antibiotic?'

Patient group	Antibiotic choice
No risk factors or atypical organisms	Flucloxacillin 2g qds IV Consider gentamicin IV If penicillin allergic use Clindamycin 450–600 mg qds IV
High risk of Gram-negative sepsis (elderly, frail, recurrent UTI and recent abdominal surgery)	Cefuroxime 1.5g tds IV Consider flucloxacillin 1g qds IV If patient penicillin allergic discuss with microbiology
MRSA risk	Vancomycin IV plus a second or third generation cephalosporin IV (e.g. cefuroxime)
Suspected gonococcus or meningococcus	Ceftriaxone IV
IV drug users ITU patients Known colonisation of other organs (e.g. patients with cystic fibrosis)	Discuss with microbiology

Figure 4.5. Recommendations for initial antibiotic therapy in septic arthritis.

- Only prescribe antibiotics for the number of days necessary to treat, i.e. usually five days for simple infections.
- Educate your patients – they don't always need an antibiotic. It is your job to educate them as to why this is the case.
- Ensure patients finish the course.

Following these very simple rules can help reduce antibiotic resistance. With changes to legislation pertaining to prescribing and the British National Formulary (BNF) being opened up to nurses, the spotlight will be on nurse prescribers. Antibiotic prescribing practice will be carefully monitored. It is your responsibility to ensure that your patients only ever get an antibiotic when it is needed, that the minimum course necessary to treat is prescribed and that your patients are educated to know that they must complete the course.

REFERENCES

Bayer AS, Taubert KA, Steckelberg J, Levison M, Dajani AS, Newburger JW et al. (1998) *Diagnosis and Management of Infective Endocarditis and Its Complications.* American Heart Association Scientific Statement. Circulation 98: 2936–48.

British Infection Society supported by the Meningitis Research Foundation (2003) Early management of suspected bacterial meningitis and meningococcal septicaemia in immunocompetent adults. *Journal of Infection* 6(2).

Coakley G et al. (2006) BSR & BHPR, BOA, RCGP and BSAC guidelines for management of hot swollen joint in adults. *Rheumatology* 45: 1039–41.

De Gan J and Van de Beek D (2002) Dexamethasone in adults with bacterial meningitis. *New England Journal of Medicine* 347: 1549–56.

Dellinger RP, Carlet JM and Masur H et al. (2004) Surviving Sepsis Campaign guidelines for management of severe sepsis and septic shock. *Critical Care Medicine* 32: 858–73.

Department of Health (1998) *The Path of Least Resistance. A Report by the Standing Medical Advisory Committee Sub-Group on Anti-Microbial Resistance*. London: DoH.

Durack DT, Lukes AS and Bright DK (1994) New criteria for diagnosis of infective endocarditis: utilization of specific echocardiographic findings: Duke Endocarditis Service. *American Journal of Medicine* 96: 200–9.

Kumar P and Clark M (2003) *Clinical Medicine*, 3rd edn. London: Saunders.

Melzer M and Pasvol G (2002) Fever in the returned traveller. *Acute Medicine Journal* 1(1): 9–14.

Spira AM (2003) Assessment of travellers who return home ill. *Lancet* 361: 1459–69.

5 Respiratory Conditions

Shortness of breath is one of the most common presenting conditions to the Medical Assessment Unit. Not being able to get one's breath is frightening and prompt assessment and management are required. The most common respiratory causes of shortness of breath are covered in this chapter.

ASTHMA

According to a National Asthma Campaign audit of 2001, 1,500 people die every year in the United Kingdom as a result of an exacerbation of asthma, which is the equivalent of four people every day. Ninety per cent of these deaths could have been prevented.

DEFINITION

Ashma is a chronic inflammatory disorder of the airways. In susceptible individuals, inflammatory symptoms are usually associated with widespread but variable airflow obstruction and an increase in airway response to a variety of stimuli. Obstruction is often reversible either spontaneously or with treatment (British Thorax Society 2003).

Asthma can be classified according to its severity. Each classification has clear criteria outlined by the British Thoracic Society guidelines for asthma management (2003). The following information is reproduced with the kind permission of the British Thoracic Society.

Near Fatal Asthma

• raised $PaCO_2$ and/or requiring mechanical ventilation with raised inflation pressures

Life-Threatening Asthma

Any one of the following in patients with severe asthma:

• Peak Expiratory Flow (PEF) <33% of best or predicted
• SpO_2 <92%
• PaO_2 <8 kPa
• normal $PaCO_2$

- silent chest
- cyanosis
- feeble respiratory effort
- bradycardia
- dysrhythmia
- hypotension
- exhaustion
- confusion
- coma

Acute Severe Asthma

- PEF 33–50% of best or predicted
- respiratory rate $\geq$25 per minute
- heart rate $\geq$110 beats/minute
- inability to complete sentences in one breath

Moderate Asthma Exacerbation

- increased symptoms
- PEF >50–75% of best or predicted
- no features of acute severe asthma

Brittle Asthma

- Type 1: wide PEF variability (>40% diurnal variation for >50% of the time over more than 150 days despite intensive therapy)
- Type 2: sudden severe attacks on a background of apparently well controlled asthma

ASSESSMENT

The British Thoracic Society has devised flow charts for the assessment of patients with exacerbation of asthma presenting to the Emergency Department. These guidelines should be utilised for all patient presenting to the Medical Assessment Unit with an exacerbation of asthma (see Figure 5.1).

When following the BTS guidelines it remains advisable to use a structured ABCDE approach in your assessment.

Airway

- Assess and maintain airway.
- Utilise head tilt, chin lift if necessary.
- Use airway adjuncts if required.

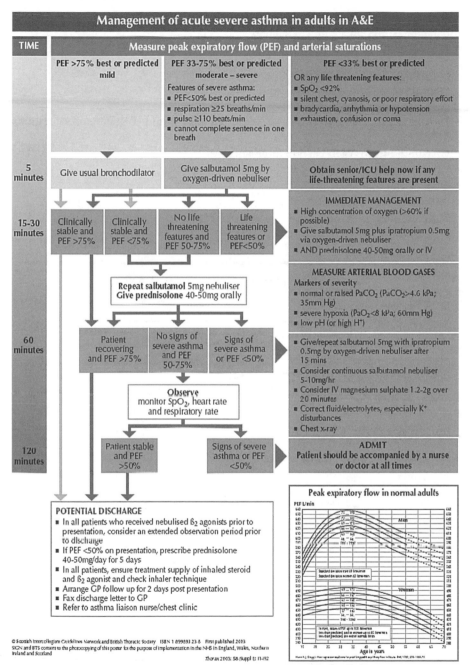

Figure 5.1. Management of acute severe asthma in adults in A&E. Reproduced with kind permission of the British Thoracic Society.

- Consider urgent referral to anaesthetist for intubation if unable to protect airway or patient has life-threatening or acute severe asthma.
- If airway compromised or patient has symptoms and signs of life-threatening or acute severe asthma, ensure medical assistance is summoned immediately.

Breathing

- Assess oxygen saturations using pulse oximeter – aim to maintain saturations at >92%.
- Give high flow oxygen via non re-breath mask.
- Consider assisting breathing with bag-valve-mask ventilation.
- Obtain arterial blood gases to assess PaO_2 and $PaCO_2$.
- Assess respiratory rate.
- If patient is able, record Peak Expiratory Flow and document patients best or predicted PEF (see Figure 5.2).

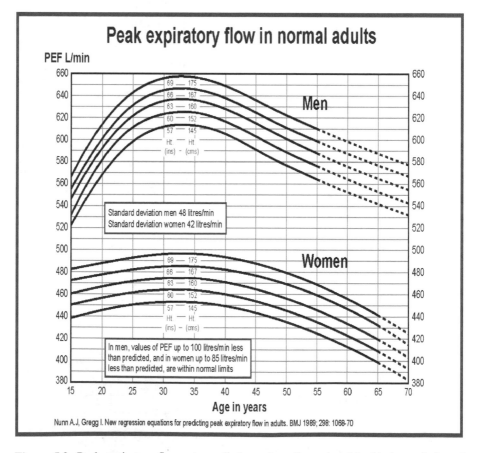

Figure 5.2. Peak expiratory flow rate predictive values. Reproduced by kind permission of BMJ Publishing Group.

- Examine respiratory system – look for signs of:
  - ➢ cyanosis
  - ➢ symmetry of movement
  - ➢ recession of intercostal spaces
  - ➢ equal chest movement
  - ➢ tracheal deviation.
- Listen for:
  - ➢ wheeze
  - ➢ decreased air entry
  - ➢ silent chest.
- Give nebulised bronchodilators via oxygen – salbutamol 5 mg and ipratropium 500 mcg.
- Give prednisolone 40 mg orally or hydrocortisone 100 mg IV 6 hourly.
- Request chest x-ray to exclude pneumothorax and consolidation.

Circulation

- Assess heart rate and rhythm.
- Record blood pressure.
- Obtain ECG.
- Gain IV access and consider administering IV magnesium sulphate 2 g over 20 minutes.
- Obtain venous blood for U&E, FBC.
- If venous potassium level is low, give IV fluids with supplemented potassium.

Disability

- Assess conscious level using AVPU.
- A deteriorating level of consciousness may be the first sign that the patient is in extremis and requires immediate medical assistance and referral to ICU.

Exposure

- Once the patient is stable a detailed, structured history and examination can be undertaken.

CHRONIC OBSTRUCTIVE PULMONARY DISEASE (COPD)

DEFINITION

COPD is a disease characterised by airflow obstruction that is not fully reversible. Airflow limitation is usually progressive and associated with an abnormal inflammatory response of the lungs to noxious particles and gases. Severity of COPD is classified into four stages. These are:

Stage 0 – At Risk

- chronic cough and sputum production
- lung function is normal

Stage I – Mild COPD

- Forced Expiratory Volume in 1 second (FEV1) $\geq$80%
- mild airflow limitation
- chronic cough and sputum production

Stage II – Moderate COPD

- FEV1 <80%
- worsening airflow limitation
- progression of symptoms
- shortness of breath on exertion

Stage III – Severe COPD

- FEV1 <30%
- severe airflow limitation
- respiratory failure
- clinical signs of right heart failure
- quality of life impaired
- exacerbations may be life threatening

SYMPTOMS AND SIGNS

Patients with an exacerbation of COPD may present with the following:

- increased shortness of breath
- wheeze
- chest tightness
- increased cough and sputum production
- pyrexia
- malaise and fatigue
- confusion
- decreased exercise tolerance

LIFE-THREATENING FEATURES

- no improvement in condition/response to treatment
- confusion
- lethargy
- coma
- worsening hypoxaemia

RESPIRATORY CONDITIONS

ASSESSMENT

The National Institute for Clinical Excellence (NICE
the management of COPD. While much of this guideli
COPD and the continuing care of patients with COPD
discussed. The guideline can be found at www.nice.o
As always, follow an ABCDE approach to assessm

Airway

- Assess and maintain airway.
- Utilise head tilt, chin lift if necessary.
- Use airway adjuncts if required.
- Consider urgent referral to anaesthetist if airway becomes compromised.

Breathing

- Assess oxygen saturations via pulse oximeter.
- Obtain arterial blood gases to assess pH, $PaCO_2$ and PaO_2.
- If arterial pH < 7.2, patient may benefit from non-invasive ventilation (NIV) and referral should be made in accordance with local policy.
- Give controlled oxygen therapy with the aim of maintaining oxygen saturations > 92%.
- Close monitoring of $PaCO_2$ will be required as some patients with COPD retain CO_2.
- Oxygen therapy should be titrated in accordance with CO_2 levels.
- Give nebulised salbutamol 5 mg and ipratropium 500 mcg via air.
- Give prednisolone 30 mg orally or hydrocortisone 100 mg IV six hourly.
- Record temperature.
- Examine respiratory system – look for signs of:
  - cyanosis
  - clubbing
  - pursed lip breathing
  - symmetry of movement
  - recession of intercostal spaces
  - equal chest movement
  - tracheal deviation.
- Listen for:
  - wheeze
  - crackles
  - decreased air entry
  - silent chest.
- Obtain CXR – assess for:
  - pneumothorax
  - consolidation
  - signs of heart failure.

of infection is present the most common bacterial pathogens are:

coccus pneumoniae

mophilus influenzae

moraxella catarrhalis.

Circulation

- Assess heart rate and rhythm.
- Record blood pressure.
- Obtain ECG.
- Gain IV access.
- Obtain venous blood for U&E, FBC.
- If venous potassium level is low, give IV fluids with supplemented potassium.
- Ensure strict fluid balance is recorded.
- Consider the need for prophylactic subcutaneous heparin or low molecular weight heparin.

Disability

- Assess conscious level using AVPU.
- A deteriorating level of consciousness may be the first sign that the patient is in extremis and requires immediate medical assistance and referral to ICU or NIV.

Exposure

- Once the patient is stable a detailed, structured history and examination can be undertaken.

PULMONARY EMBOLISM

Pulmonary embolism (PE) is often missed clinically. It should be suspected in any patient with vague symptoms, in those who are not responding to initial therapy and in any case of unexplained clinical deterioration (British Thoracic Society 2003).

Most cases of PE follow a popliteal or ileofemoral deep vein thrombosis (DVT).

As a rule patients with small emboli present with dyspnoea and those with a moderate-sized embolism present with pleuritic chest pain and signs of infarction.

PE can be fatal, therefore prompt recognition and assessment is required.

SYMPTOMS AND SIGNS

As already stated symptoms can be vague and signs may be absent. Clinical suspicion is paramount and pre-test probability can be assessed by following a simple flow chart (see Figure 5.3).

Some of the more common symptoms and signs are:

- dyspnoea – may be sudden onset and is present in 90% of cases
- pleuritic chest pain
- haemoptysis
- syncope
- tachycardia – heart rate >100 beats/min
- tachypnoea – respirations >20/min
- fever

Clinical features	
Score points as shown for each of the following features	
Symptoms of DVT with objective swelling of leg and pain on palpation over deep vein	3.0
Heart rate >100 beats per minute	1.5
Bedrest for >3 consecutive days or surgery in past 4 weeks	1.5
Previous confirmed DVT or PE	1.5
Haemoptysis	1.0
Cancer treated within previous 6 months or patient receiving palliative care	1.0
PE as likely or more likely than alternative diagnosis, taking into account clinical features, chest x-ray and ECG	3.0
Total score	Pre-test probability
<2.0	Low
2.0–6.0	Moderate
>6.0	High

Figure 5.3. Clinical scoring table for PE.

LIFE-THREATENING FEATURES

Features consistent with a massive PE require immediate medical assistance. If a patient presents with features of a massive PE summon help immediately.

Features of massive PE are:

- severe dyspnoea
- dull central chest pain
- elevated venous pressure
- evidence of right-sided heart failure
- hypotension
- shock

ASSESSMENT

The British Thoracic Society issued guidance on the assessment and management of patients with suspected PE in 2003. The full guideline can be found at www.brit-thoracic.org.uk

As always, utilise an ABCDE approach to assessment.

Airway

- Assess and maintain airway.
- Utilise head tilt, chin lift if necessary.
- Use airway adjuncts if required.
- Consider urgent referral to anaesthetist for intubation if unable to protect airway.

Breathing

- Assess oxygen saturations using pulse oximeter – aim to maintain saturations at >92%.
- Give high flow oxygen via non re-breath mask.
- Consider assisting breathing with bag-valve-mask ventilation.
- Obtain arterial blood gases to assess PaO_2 and $PaCO_2$.
- Assess respiratory rate.
- Examine respiratory system.
- Listen for a pleuritic rub.
- Request chest x-ray – this may be normal, but look for:
  - ➢ evidence of wedge shaped shadow (infarct)
  - ➢ linear atelectasis
  - ➢ pleural effusion
  - ➢ raised hemidiaphragm.
- If clinical suspicion is high following assessment, request a ventilation perfusion scan (VQ) or CT Pulmonary Angiogram (CTPA) in accordance with local protocols.

Circulation

- Assess heart rate and rhythm – a right ventricular heave may be felt and the second heart sound accentuated with a gallop rhythm.
- Assess JVP – this may be raised.
- Record blood pressure.
- Obtain ECG – may show:
  - ➢ sinus tachycardia
  - ➢ S1 Q3 T3 pattern
  - ➢ right bundle branch block
  - ➢ right axis deviation
  - ➢ p pulmonale.
- Gain IV access.
- Obtain venous blood for U&E, FBC, INR and D-dimer.
- If PE suspected commence subcutaneous low molecular weight heparin.
- If life-threatening features are present expert help is required as thrombolysis may be indicated.
- If patient is for thrombolysis, alteplase is the recommended drug of choice. Give 50 mg IV as a bolus injection.

- It patient fails to respond to thrombolysis, urgent referral to a specialist for thromboembolectomy is indicated and this should be done in accordance with local protocols.

Disability

- Assess conscious level using AVPU.
- A deteriorating level of consciousness may be the first sign that the patient is in extremis and requires immediate medical assistance and referral to ICU.

Exposure

- Always assess the pre-test probability for PE (Figure 5.3), taking into account risk factors and results from initial ABCDE assessment.
- Once the patient is stable a detailed, structured history and examination can be undertaken.
- Don't forget to examine for signs of DVT.

RISK FACTORS FOR PE

- DVT – this is present in 50% of patients
- recent surgery
- recent trauma
- immobility for any reason
- malignancy
- patients taking the oral contraceptive pill
- patients on hormone replacement therapy
- late pregnancy
- obesity
- patients taking Selective Estregen Receptor Modulator therapy (SERM)
- hyperviscosity syndromes
- pureperium
- nephrotic syndrome
- defective fibrinolysis
- antithrombin III deficiency
- protein C and protein S deficiency
- lupus anticoagulant

TREATMENT FOR CONFIRMED PE

Once a PE has been diagnosed by VQ scan or CTPA it is necessary to start anticoagulation therapy. Low molecular weight heparin will have already been commenced prior to the requisite scans being undertaken. This must continue until INR is within therapeutic range with warfarin for two consecutive days.

The duration of treatment with warfarin will depend on the individual patient's history. Patient's in whom the PE is a first event should be considered for anticoagulation for 3–6 months. For those in whom this is a recurrent event, lifelong warfarin will be required.

Fennerty et al. (1984) devised a method of initiating anticoagulation to gain therapeutic control as quickly as possible. It is recommended that this regime is used when initiating patients on to warfarin (Figure 5.4).

Before commencing warfarin, patients should be counselled, ideally by a pharmacist trained in this role, as to the dos and don'ts when taking warfarin.

Occasionally it can take longer than expected to gain therapeutic control of INR. If a patient requires Low Molecular Weight Heparin for longer than one week platelet levels must be checked every seven days. While this is not the remit of the practitioner in the Medical Assessment Unit this should be documented in the patient's medical notes for the admitting ward.

COMMUNITY AND HOSPITAL ACQUIRED PNEUMONIA

Community acquired pneumonia is more likely to be seen in the Medical Assessment Unit than hospital acquired pneumonia. Hospital acquired pneumonia is pneumonia presenting >48 hours after admission to hospital and excluding infection that was incubating at the time of admission to hospital. The only time hospital acquired pneumonia may be seen in MAU is following a patient being re-admitted within 48 hours of discharge from hospital. Assessment of patients with all types of pneumonia remains identical, it is the antibiotic therapy that may differ, depending on local policies for antibiotic therapy.

DEFINITION

Pneumonia is defined as an inflammation of the substance of the lungs. This is usually caused by bacteria. Pneumonia can be classified according to where it occurs anatomically or the basis of its aetiology.

Anatomical Classifications

- lobar pneumonia – affecting the whole of one lobe
- bronchopneumonia – affecting the lobules and bronchi

Aetiological Classifications

- community acquired pneumonia
- hospital acquired pneumonia
- aspiration pneumonia
- pneumonia in the immunosuppressed

Day 1	
INR	**Warfarin dose (mg)**
<1.4	10.0
≥ 1.4	This predictive method cannot be used. Choice of dose must rely on clinical judgement
Day 2 (16 hours after 1st dose)	
INR	**Warfarin dose (mg)**
<1.8	10.0
1.8	1.0
>1.8	0.5
Day 3 (16 hours after 2nd dose)	
INR	**Warfarin dose (mg)**
<2.0	10.0
2.0–2.1	5.0
2.2–2.3	4.5
2.4–2.5	4.0
2.6–2.7	3.5
2.8–2.9	3.0
3.0–3.1	2.5
3.2–3.3	2.0
3.4	1.5
3.5	1.0
3.6 .0	0.5
>4.0	0
Day 4 (16 hours after 3rd dose)	
INR	**Warfarin dose (mg)**
<1.4	>8.0
1.4	8.0
1.5	7.5
1.6–1.7	7.0
1.8	6.5
1.9	6.0
2.0–2.1	5.5
2.2–2.3	5.0
2.4–2.6	4.5
2.7–3.0	4.0
3.1–3.5	3.5
3.6–4.0	3.0
4.1–4.5	0 – give 2 mg from day 5
>4.5	0 – give 1 mg from day 6

The dose selected on day 4 is the predicted maintenance dose necessary to achieve a stable INR in the range 2–4.

Figure 5.4. Predictive method for warfarin loading. *Source*: Fennerty et al. (1984) Reproduced with kind permission of BMJ Publishing Group.

SYMPTOMS AND SIGNS

Common presenting symptoms of patients with pneumonia are:

- fever
- rigors
- malaise
- shortness of breath and tachypnoea
- cough and sputum production
- vomiting
- diarrhoea
- pleuritic chest pain
- tachycardia

LIFE-THREATENING FEATURES

Patients with any of the following signs require urgent referral to ICU. Summon medical assistance immediately.

- arterial PaO_2 ≤ 8 kPa with an inspired O_2 $\geq 60\%$
- severe acidosis – pH < 7.25
- exhaustion
- drowsiness
- unconscious patient
- signs of shock

ASSESSMENT

The British Thoracic Society issued guidelines for the management of community acquired pneumonia in 2001 and these were updated in 2004. They are reflected in the following guidance.

As always, utilise an ABCDE approach to assessment.

Airway

- Assess and maintain airway.
- Utilise head tilt, chin lift if necessary.
- Use airway adjuncts if required.
- Consider urgent referral to anaesthetist for intubation if unable to protect airway.

Breathing

- Assess oxygen saturations using pulse oximeter – aim to maintain saturations at $> 92\%$.
- Give high flow oxygen via non re-breath mask to maintain SaO_2 at $> 92\%$.

- Obtain arterial blood gases if SaO_2 <92% to assess PaO_2 and $PaCO_2$.
- Assess respiratory rate.
- Examine respiratory system – listen for:
  - ➢ localised crackles
  - ➢ bronchial breathing
  - ➢ pleural rub may be present.
- Request chest x-ray – this may be normal as changes lag behind the clinical course but look for:
  - ➢ consolidation
  - ➢ pleural effusion.
- Obtain sputum for microscopy, culture and sensitivity.

Circulation

- Assess heart rate and rhythm.
- Record blood pressure.
- Obtain ECG.
- Gain IV access.
- Obtain venous blood for U&E, FBC, LFTs and CRP.
- Obtain blood cultures.
- Prescribe IV fluids (normal saline or dextrose saline over 6–8 hours) as the patient is likely to be slightly dehydrated. This can be adjusted once U&E results are known.
- Ensure strict fluid balance is maintained.
- If pleuritic pain is present, give analgesia – a non-steroidal may be best if there are no contraindications.

Disability

- Assess conscious level using AVPU.
- A deteriorating level of consciousness may be the first sign that the patient is in extremis and requires immediate medical assistance and referral to ICU.
- Assess severity of pneumonia using the CURB-65 score (British Thoracic Society 2001, updated 2004).

CURB-65 Score*

All patients with community acquired pneumonia admitted to hospital should be assessed following these criteria. Score 1 point for each sign that is present.

- Confusion
- Urea >7 mmol/l
- Respiratory rate ≥30 breaths/min

* Permission to reproduce the Curb-65 Score has been granted by the British Thoracic Society.

- **B**lood pressure systolic <90 mmHg or diastolic ≤60 mmHg
- Age ≥**65** years

The total score indicates the risk of death to the patient.

- Score 0–1 = low risk of death – likely suitable for home treatment.
- Score 2 = some increased risk of death – consider hospital supervised treatment.
- Score ≥3 = high risk of death – requires urgent medical assessment and consideration for ICU admission, especially if CURB-65 score is 4 or 5.

Once the patient has been assessed following ABCD, and treatment has been commenced, don't forget to complete your assessment with E for Exposure.

Exposure

- Once the patient is stable, a detailed, structured history and examination can be undertaken.

ANTIBIOTIC TREATMENT

As covered in Chapter 4 antibiotic policies vary, depending on local patterns of sensitivity and resistance. It is therefore imperative that you familiarise yourself with local antibiotic guidelines.

The route of administration will depend on the patient's ability to swallow, the severity of the pneumonia and the likely pathogen. Antibiotic treatment should be commenced as soon as a diagnosis of pneumonia is made. Do not wait for the results of blood and sputum culture. Whatever therapy is chosen, the antibiotic to be administered should always cover the pathogen streptococcus pneumoniae.

Suggestions for antibiotic treatment:

- Non-severe community acquired pneumonia:
  - ➢ amoxicillin 500 mg 8 hourly (tds) **or**
  - ➢ moxifloxacin 400 mg once daily **or**
  - ➢ erythromycin 500 mg 6 hourly (qds).
- Severe community acquired pneumonia:
  - ➢ moxifloxacin 400 mg once daily **plus**
  - ➢ benzylpenicillin 1.2 g IV 6 hourly **or**
  - ➢ levofloxacin 500 mg IV daily.

PNEUMOTHORAX

DEFINITION

Pneumothorax is the presence of air in the pleural space. A pneumothorax can occur spontaneously or as a result of trauma (British Thoracic Society 2003). A tension pneumothorax is a result of positive pressure building up when air passes into the pleura on inspiration. This can lead to cardiorespiratory distress and cardiac arrest. Tension pneumothorax is rare but spontaneous pneumothorax is a common cause of admission to MAU.

SYMPTOMS AND SIGNS

Patients with a spontaneous pneumothorax present with the following:

- chest pain – usually only on the affected side
- shortness of breath
- tachycardia

LIFE-THREATENING FEATURES

- patient in extremis – consider possible tension pneumothorax
- acutely short of breath
- hypotension
- tachycardia
- tracheal displacement

ASSESSMENT

As always, utilise an ABCDE approach to assessment.

Airway

- Assess and maintain airway.
- Utilise head tilt, chin lift if necessary.
- Use airway adjuncts if required.
- Consider urgent referral to anaesthetist for intubation if unable to protect airway.

Breathing

- Assess oxygen saturations using pulse oximeter – aim to maintain saturations at >92%.
- Give high-flow oxygen via non re-breath mask.
- Consider assisting breathing with bag-valve-mask ventilation.
- Obtain arterial blood gases to assess PaO_2 and $PaCO_2$.
- Assess respiratory rate.
- Examine respiratory system.
- Look for signs of tracheal deviation – if deviated suspect tension pneumothorax:
  - ➢ summon medical help immediately.
  - ➢ insert large bore cannula into the second intercostal space in the mid clavicular line.
  - ➢ a chest drain will need to be inserted once patient is stable.

- request PA chest x-ray. This will determine your course of action:
  - ➤ if CXR reveals small collapse with <2 cm rim of air and patient is not significantly short of breath and does not have chronic lung disease – observe for four hours and then consider discharge
  - ➤ if CXR reveals small collapse with <2 cm rim of air and patient has chronic lung disease – admit for overnight observation and consider discharge the following day
  - ➤ if CXR reveals small collapse with <2 cm rim of air and patient is significantly short of breath – consider aspiration of the pneumothorax and overnight observation in hospital
  - ➤ if CXR reveals a pneumothorax with a rim of air ≥2 cm, the patient requires admission and insertion of an intercostal drain – seek medical support.

Circulation

- Assess heart rate and rhythm.
- Record blood pressure.
- Obtain ECG.
- Gain IV access.
- Obtain venous blood for U&E and FBC.

Disability

- Assess conscious level using AVPU.
- A deteriorating level of consciousness may be the first sign that the patient is in extremis and requires immediate medical assistance and referral to ICU.

Exposure

- Once the patient is stable, a detailed, structured history and examination can be undertaken.

TYPE I RESPIRATORY FAILURE

DEFINITION

Type I respiratory failure is defined as hypoxia (PaO_2 <8 kPa) with a normal or low $PaCO_2$.

Type I respiratory failure can be due to a number of conditions:

- asthma
- COPD
- pneumonia
- pulmonary oedema
- Acute Respiratory Distress Syndrome (ARDS)

- fibrosing alveolitis
- right-to-left cardiac shunts
- pneumothorax
- pulmonary embolism

SYMPTOMS AND SIGNS

Patients with Type I respiratory failure present with the following:

- tachypnoea
- tachycardia
- sweating
- cyanosis
- use of accessory muscles
- pulsus paradoxus

ASSESSMENT

As always, follow an ABCDE approach to assessment.

Airway

- Assess and maintain airway.
- Utilise head tilt, chin lift if necessary.
- Use airway adjuncts if required.
- Consider urgent referral to anaesthetist if airway becomes compromised.

Breathing

- Assess oxygen saturations via pulse oximeter.
- Obtain arterial blood gases to assess pH, $PaCO_2$ and PaO_2.
- Give oxygen therapy with the aim of maintaining oxygen saturations >92% and PaO_2 >8 kPa.
- If PaO_2 remains <8 kPa despite high flow oxygen refer urgently to an anaesthetist for possible assisted ventilation
- Give nebulised salbutamol 5 mg and ipratropium 500 mcg if patient is wheezy.
- Record temperature.
- Examine respiratory system – look for signs of:
  - cyanosis
  - clubbing
  - pursed lip breathing
  - symmetry of movement
  - recession of intercostal spaces
  - equal chest movement
  - tracheal deviation.

- Listen for:
  - ➢ wheeze
  - ➢ crackles
  - ➢ decreased air entry
  - ➢ silent chest.
- Obtain CXR – assess for:
  - pneumothorax
  - consolidation
  - signs of heart failure.
- Arterial blood gases will need to be repeated in order to assess effectiveness of oxygen therapy.

Circulation

- Assess heart rate and rhythm.
- Record blood pressure.
- Obtain ECG.
- Gain IV access.
- Obtain venous blood for U&E, FBC.
- If venous potassium level is low, give IV fluids with supplemented potassium.
- Ensure strict fluid balance is recorded.
- Consider the need for prophylactic subcutaneous heparin or Low Molecular Weight Heparin.

Disability

- Assess conscious level using AVPU.
- A deteriorating level of consciousness may be the first sign that the patient is in extremis and requires immediate medical assistance and referral to ICU.

Exposure

- Once the patient is stable, a detailed, structured history and examination can be undertaken.
- Ensure the underlying cause of respiratory failure is appropriately and adequately treated.

TYPE II RESPIRATORY FAILURE

DEFINITION

Type II respiratory failure is defined as hypoxia (PaO_2 <8 kPa) with hypercapnia ($PaCO_2$ >6.5 kPa).

Type II respiratory failure can be due to a number of conditions:

- COPD
- severe asthma
- neuromuscular disorders
- respiratory depression due to medication
- chest wall deformities
- muscular dystrophies
- encephalitis

Symptoms and Signs

Patients with Type II respiratory failure present with the following:

- tachypnoea
- tachycardia
- sweating
- use of accessory muscles
- cyanosis
- bounding pulse
- coarse tremor
- warm peripheries
- papilloedema
- drowsiness

ASSESSMENT

As always, follow an ABCDE approach to assessment.

Airway

- Assess and maintain airway.
- Utilise head tilt, chin lift if necessary.
- Use airway adjuncts if required.
- Consider urgent referral to anaesthetist if airway becomes compromised.

Breathing

- Assess oxygen saturations via pulse oximeter.
- Obtain arterial blood gases to assess pH, $PaCO_2$ and PaO_2.
- Give oxygen therapy cautiously. Start with 24% oxygen.
- The aim of oxygen therapy is to maintain oxygen saturations >92% and PaO_2 >6.5 kPa.
- Repeat ABGs after 20 minutes.
- If $PaCO_2$ remains unchanged or has risen, increase oxygen therapy to 28%.

- If PaCO$_2$ has risen by >1 kPa and the patient remains hypoxic, consider the use of a respiratory stimulant such as IV Doxapram.
- If you have not already done so get medical assistance now.
- If patient continues to retain CO$_2$ and remains hypoxic, referral for possible NIV should be considered.
- Every time oxygen therapy is adjusted, ABGs should be repeated after 20–30 minutes to assess effectiveness of treatment.
- Record temperature.
- Examine respiratory system – look for signs of:
  - cyanosis
  - clubbing
  - pursed lip breathing
  - symmetry of movement
  - recession of intercostal spaces
  - equal chest movement
  - tracheal deviation.
- Listen for:
  - wheeze
  - crackles
  - decreased air entry
  - silent chest.
- Obtain CXR – assess for:
  - pneumothorax
  - consolidation
  - signs of heart failure.

Circulation

- Assess heart rate and rhythm.
- Record blood pressure.
- Obtain ECG.
- Gain IV access.
- Obtain venous blood for U&E, FBC.
- If venous potassium level is low, give IV fluids with supplemented potassium.
- Ensure strict fluid balance is recorded.
- Consider the need for prophylactic subcutaneous heparin or low molecular weight heparin.

Disability

- Assess conscious level using AVPU.
- A deteriorating level of consciousness may be the first sign that the patient is in extremis and requires immediate medical assistance and referral to ICU.

Exposure

- Once the patient is stable, a detailed, structured history and examination can be undertaken.
- Ensure the underlying cause of respiratory failure is appropriately and adequately treated.

REFERENCES

British Thoracic Society (2001, updated 2004) Guidelines for the management of community acquired pneumonia. *Thorax* 86, suppl. IV.

British Thoracic Society (2002) Non-invasive ventilation in acute respiratory failure. *Thorax* 57: 192–211.

British Thoracic Society (2003) Guidelines for the management of suspected acute pulmonary embolism. British Thoracic Society Standards of Care Committee Pulmonary Embolism Guideline Development Group. *Thorax* 58: 470–84.

BTS/SIGN (2003) British guideline on the management of asthma. *Thorax* 38, suppl. 1.

Fennerty A, Dolben J and Thomas P (1984) Flexible induction dose regimen for warfarin and predictive maintenance dose. *British Medical Journal* 288: 1268–70.

Henry M, Arnold T and Harvey J (2003) British Thoracic Society Guidelines for the management of spontaneous pneumothorax. *Thorax* 58, suppl. 2: 39–52.

National Institute for Clinical Excellence (2004) *Chronic Obstructive Pulmonary Disease. Management of chronic obstructive pulmonary disease in primary and secondary care.* Clinical Guideline 12. London: NICE.

6 Cardiovascular Conditions

Ischaemic heart disease is the leading cause of death in the world. In Europe, cardiovascular disease accounts for approximately 40% of all deaths in people under the age of 75 years. With this in mind it is important that patients presenting with cardiovascular conditions are assessed and treated promptly.

ACUTE CORONARY SYNDROMES (ACS)

DEFINITION

Acute coronary syndromes cover a spectrum of conditions. This group comprises:

- unstable angina
- non-ST segment elevation myocardial infarction (NSTEMI)
- ST segment elevation myocardial infarction (STEMI)

The disease process that occurs is:

- Haemorrhage into the plaque. This causes it to swell and restrict the lumen of the artery.
- Contraction of the smooth muscle within the artery wall. This causes further constriction of the lumen.
- Thrombus formation on the surface of the plaque. This may cause partial or complete obstruction of the lumen of the artery.

It is the extent to which blood flow to the myocardium is reduced as a result of these events that determines the nature of the ensuing ACS.

STABLE ANGINA

SIGNS AND SYMPTOMS

Signs and symptoms for all ACS are frequently the same. Common presenting complaints are:

- Pain in chest – described as:
  - ➢ a tightness
  - ➢ indigestion like pain

- ➢ crushing
- ➢ a band around chest
- ➢ 'like someone sitting on my chest'.
- Pain may radiate down the left arm, both arms and/or into the jaw.
- Pain may be accompanied by:
  - ➢ sweating
  - ➢ shortness of breath
  - ➢ nausea and vomiting.

Stable angina is angina pain that only occurs on exercise and settles quickly on resting. This is not classified as an ACS and hopefully should not be seen in MAU.

UNSTABLE ANGINA

In contrast to stable angina, unstable angina is defined by the occurrence of one or more of the following:

- Angina on exertion occurring over a period of a few days and increasing in frequency. Progressively less exertion is required to provoke an episode of angina. This is commonly called 'crescendo angina'.
- Episodes of angina occurring recurrently and unpredictably. They are not specifically provoked by exercise. They are frequently short lived and may settle spontaneously or be temporarily relieved by sub-lingual glyceryl trinitrate (GTN).
- An unprovoked and prolonged episode of chest pain. No definite evidence of myocardial infarction.

The Resuscitation Council UK (2005) have issued guidance on the management of patients with ACS. This is supported by the National Service Framework for Coronary Heart Disease (2000).

SIGNS AND SYMPTOMS
- Pain in chest – described as:
  - ➢ a tightness
  - ➢ indigestion like pain
  - ➢ crushing
  - ➢ a band around the chest
  - ➢ 'like someone sitting on my chest'.
- Pain may radiate down the left arm, both arms and/or into the jaw.
- Pain may be accompanied by:
  - ➢ sweating
  - ➢ shortness of breath
  - ➢ nausea and vomiting.

ASSESSMENT

Prompt recognition and assessment is vital. As always, follow an ABCDE approach to assessment.

Airway

- Assess and maintain airway.
- Utilise head tilt, chin lift if necessary.
- Use airway adjuncts if required.
- Consider urgent referral to anaesthetist for intubation if unable to protect airway.

Breathing

- Assess oxygen saturations using pulse oximeter – aim to maintain saturations at >92%.
- Give high flow oxygen via non re-breath mask.
- Consider assisting breathing with bag-valve-mask ventilation.
- Assess respiratory rate.
- Examine respiratory system.
- Request chest x-ray.

Circulation

- Assess heart rate and rhythm.
- Record blood pressure.
- Obtain ECG – may be normal but ST depression is common.
- Gain IV access.
- Obtain venous blood for U&E, FBC, cardiac enzymes or Troponin depending on local protocols (enzymes and Troponin should not be elevated in unstable angina).
- Remember MONA:
  - ➢ Morphine – give 5 mg IV
  - ➢ Oxygen – high flow
  - ➢ Nitrate – give sublingual GTN
  - ➢ Aspirin – give 300 mg as a stat dose even if already on aspirin.
- Give low molecular weight heparin until the patient has been pain free for 24 hours.
- Consider adding clopidogrel, 300 mg loading dose followed by maintenance of 75 mg daily.

Disability

- Assess conscious level using AVPU.

Exposure

- Once the patient is stable a detailed, structured history and examination can be undertaken.

NON-ST ELEVATION MYOCARDIAL INFARCTION

Some patients with NSTEMI are at a high risk of progressing to coronary occlusion, leading to more extensive myocardial damage and arrhythmias causing death. The risk of this occurring is greatest within the first few hours of the initial event and this risk diminishes with time.

SIGNS AND SYMPTOMS

- Pain in chest – described as:
  - ➤ a tightness
  - ➤ indigestion like pain
  - ➤ crushing
  - ➤ a band around the chest
  - ➤ 'like someone sitting on my chest'.
- Pain may radiate down the left arm, both arms and/or into the jaw.
- Pain may be accompanied by:
  - ➤ sweating
  - ➤ shortness of breath
  - ➤ nausea and vomiting.

ASSESSMENT

Prompt recognition and assessment is vital. Medical assistance should be summoned. As always, follow an ABCDE approach to assessment.

Airway

- Assess and maintain airway.
- Utilise head tilt, chin lift if necessary.
- Use airway adjuncts if required.
- Consider urgent referral to anaesthetist for intubation if unable to protect airway.

Breathing

- Assess oxygen saturations using pulse oximeter – aim to maintain saturations at >92%.
- Give high flow oxygen via non re-breath mask.
- Consider assisting breathing with bag-valve-mask ventilation.
- Assess respiratory rate.
- Examine respiratory system.
- Request chest x-ray.

Circulation

- Assess heart rate and rhythm.
- Record blood pressure.
- Obtain ECG – ST depression or T wave inversion is common.
- Gain IV access.
- Obtain venous blood for U&E, FBC, cardiac enzymes or Troponin depending on local protocols (the amount of cardiac enzyme or Troponin released indicates the degree of myocardial damage).
- Monitor blood glucose – if >11 mmol/l follow DIGAMI regime (see section after STEMI).
- Remember MONA:
  - ➤ Morphine – give 5 mg IV
  - ➤ Oxygen – high flow
  - ➤ Nitrate – give sublingual GTN
  - ➤ Aspirin – give 300 mg as a stat dose even if already on aspirin.
- Give low molecular weight heparin until the patient has been pain free for 24 hours.
- Consider adding clopidogrel, loading dose of 300 mg followed by maintenance of 75 mg daily.
- Addition of a beta blocker and statin should be considered.

Disability

- Assess conscious level using AVPU.

Exposure

- Once the patient is stable a detailed, structured history and examination can be undertaken. Following NSTEMI a patient must not drive for four weeks. While the MAU is not the appropriate place to have a conversation regarding driving, it is important that it is documented in the medical notes that the patient needs to be informed of this prior to discharge. The patient does not need to inform the DVLA.

ST ELEVATION MYOCARDIAL INFARCTION

STEMI occurs when there is an acute complete occlusion of a coronary artery. Left untreated there will be further myocardial damage. During the acute phase there is an increased risk of ventricular fibrillation or tachycardia leading to sudden death. Medical assistance should be summoned.

Signs and symptoms

- Pain in chest – described as:
  - ➤ a tightness
  - ➤ indigestion like pain

➤ crushing
➤ a band around the chest
➤ 'like someone sitting on my chest'.
• Pain may radiate down the left arm, both arms and/or into the jaw.
• Pain may be accompanied by:
➤ sweating
➤ shortness of breath
➤ nausea and vomiting.

ASSESSMENT

Prompt recognition and assessment is vital. As always, follow an ABCDE approach to assessment.

Airway

• Assess and maintain airway.
• Utilise head tilt, chin lift if necessary.
• Use airway adjuncts if required.
• Consider urgent referral to anaesthetist for intubation if unable to protect airway.

Breathing

• Assess oxygen saturations using pulse oximeter – aim to maintain saturations at >92%.
• Give high flow oxygen via non re-breath mask.
• Consider assisting breathing with bag-valve-mask ventilation.
• Assess respiratory rate.
• Examine respiratory system.
• Request chest x-ray.

Circulation

• Assess heart rate and rhythm.
• Record blood pressure.
• Obtain ECG – acute ST segment elevation or new left bundle branch block (LBBB) in conjunction with symptoms of a myocardial infarction indicate the need for reperfusion therapy.
• Typical ECG changes in STEMI are:
➤ anterior/anteroseptal – seen in V1–V4
➤ inferior – seen in II, III and aVF
➤ lateral – seen in V5–V6 and I and aVL
➤ posterior – reciprocal changes in anterior leads.

Absolute

- Previous haemorrhagic stroke.
- Ischaemic stroke during the previous 6 months.
- Central nervous system damage or neoplasm.
- Recent major surgery, head injury or other major trauma (within last 3 weeks).
- Active internal bleeding or gastro-intestinal bleeding within the past month.
- Known bleeding disorder.

Relative

- Refractory hypertension (systolic blood pressure >180 mmHg).
- Transient iscahemic attack in preceding 6 months.
- Oral anticoagulant therapy.
- Pregnancy or less than 1 week post-partum.
- Traumatic CPR.
- Non-compressible vascular puncture.
- Active peptic ulcer disease.
- Advanced liver disease.
- Infective endocarditis.
- Previous allergic reaction to the thrombolytic drug to be used.

If streptokinase has been given more than 4 days previously use a different thrombolytic agent.

Figure 6.1. Contraindications to thrombolysis therapy.

- Gain IV access.
- Obtain venous blood for U&E, FBC, cardiac enzymes or Troponin, depending on local policies
- Monitor blood glucose – if >11 mmol/l, follow DIGAMI regime (in next section).
- Remember MONA:
  - ➢ Morphine – give 5 mg IV
  - ➢ Oxygen – high flow
  - ➢ Nitrate – give sublingual GTN
  - ➢ Aspirin – give 300 mg as a stat dose even if already on aspirin.
- Assess suitability for thrombolysis (see Figure 6.1) – drugs used in thrombolysis are:
  - ➢ streptokinase – 1.5 million units in 100 mls normal saline
  - ➢ alteplase – 15 mg bolus then infusion of 0.75 mg/kg over 1 hour
  - ➢ reteplase – 10 units bolus then further 10 units after 30 minutes
  - ➢ tenecteplase – 30–50 mg (6,000–10,000 units) as a bolus.
- All these patients require urgent referral to a cardiologist.

Disability

- Assess conscious level using AVPU.

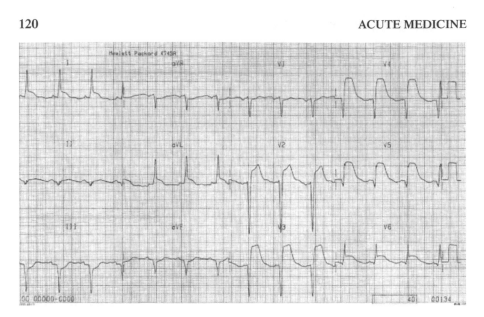

Figure 6.2. Anterolateral MI.

Exposure

- Once the patient is stable a detailed, structured history and examination can be undertaken.
- Following STEMI a patient must not drive for four weeks. While the MAU is not the appropriate place to have a conversation regarding driving it is important that it is documented in the medical notes that the patient needs to be informed of this prior to discharge. The patient does not need to inform the DVLA.

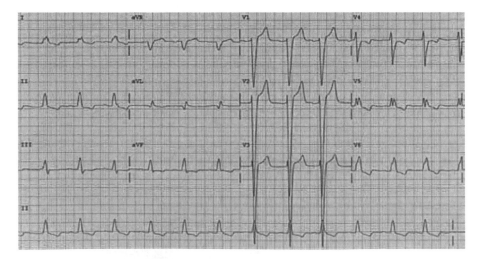

Figure 6.3. Left bundle branch block.

Capillary glucose (mmol/L)	Actrapid – rate of infusion in units per hour
>15	6
11–14.9	5
7–10.9	3
4–6.9	1
<4	Stop insulin infusion and administer 50 mls of 20% Glucose IV Monitor capillary blood glucose every 15 minutes Recommence insulin infusion when blood glucose >7 mmol/L

Figure 6.4. DIGAMI regime.

DIGAMI

The Diabetes and Insulin-Glucose infusion in Acute Myocardial Infarction (DIGAMI) study (1995) by Malmberg et al. showed that by treating hyperglycaemia following an MI with insulin for three months, outcome was improved.

It is therefore vital to record blood glucose in all MI patients and if they are found to have a blood glucose >11 mmol/l, insulin should be commenced in accordance with the following guideline:

- Record two-hourly capillary blood glucose.
- Obtain venous potassium – do not wait for the result – commence treatment and titrate once potassium level is known.
- Prepare an insulin infusion of 50 units Actrapid in 50 mls sodium chloride and commence at 4 units/hour.
- Further adjustments should be made in accordance with the information in Figure 6.4.
- Administer 5% glucose IV at a rate of 1 l every 12 hours.
- If potassium level is <4.5 mmol/l administer 5% glucose with 20 mmol potassium chloride over 12 hours.
- This regime should be continued for 24–72 hours.
- When capillary blood glucose is stable for 24 hours a basal bolus regime can be commenced (add up total insulin requirements over 24 hours and divide into four equal doses).

ARRHYTHMIAS

Cardiac arrhythmias if left untreated, can lead to a rapid deterioration in a patient's clinical condition and potentially cardiac arrest. Expert help should always be summoned promptly.

When a patient presents with a known or suspected cardiac arrhythmia you should consider two things:

- How is the patient?
- What is the rhythm?

The Resuscitation Council UK advocate a simple six-stage approach to analysing rhythms. If you are unsure of the presenting rhythm follow these six simple steps to describe what you see (reproduced with kind permission of the Resuscitation Council UK):

- Is there any electrical activity?
- What is the ventricular (QRS) rate?
- Is the QRS rhythm regular or irregular?
- Is the QRS complex normal or prolonged?
- Is atrial activity present?
- Is atrial activity related to ventricular activity and, if so, how?

For all arrhythmias, following assessment, the decision on mode of treatment will depend on the clinical condition of the patient. If the patient is stable and there are no adverse signs, there is no urgency for treatment. However, the patient with adverse signs is at high risk of deterioration and cardiac arrest and therefore requires prompt treatment.

ADVERSE SIGNS

If a patient with an arrhythmia has any of the following signs immediate referral to cardiologist or senior medical colleague is required.

- pallor
- sweating
- cold extremities
- hypotension
- drowsiness
- confusion
- excessive tachycardia – heart rate >150 beats/minute
- excessive bradycardia – heart rate <40 beats/minute
- heart failure
- chest pain

The most common arrhythmias now follow. For each presenting arrhythmia there are a number of treatment options depending on the rhythm and the patient's clinical condition. Commonly, the options are:

- no immediate treatment required
- physical manoeuvres such as vagal stimulation

- anti-arrhythmic drugs
- electrical cardioversion
- cardiac pacing

BRADYCARDIA

DEFINITION

Bradycardia is defined as a heart rate of <60 beats/minute. For some people this is not a clinical risk, as bradycardia can be as a result of, for example, fitness or drug use (beta blockers).

Extreme bradycardia is defined as:

- heart rate <40 beats/minute
- rarely well tolerated
- requires immediate treatment
- considered an adverse feature

Less severe bradycardia is defined as:

- heart rate of 40–60 beats/minute
- requires immediate treatment if adverse features are present

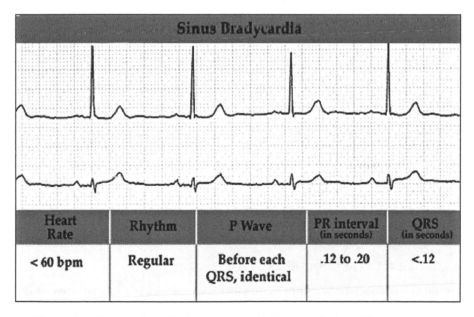

Heart Rate	Rhythm	P Wave	PR interval (in seconds)	QRS (in seconds)
< 60 bpm	Regular	Before each QRS, identical	.12 to .20	<.12

Figure 6.5. Sinus bradycardia. Reproduced with kind permission of Frank Yanowitz.

ASSESSMENT

As always, follow an ABCDE approach to assessment.

Airway

- Assess and maintain airway.
- Utilise head tilt, chin lift if necessary.
- Use airway adjuncts if required.
- Consider urgent referral to anaesthetist for intubation if unable to protect airway.

Breathing

- Assess oxygen saturations using pulse oximeter – aim to maintain saturations at >92%.
- Give high-flow oxygen via non re-breath mask.
- Assess respiratory rate.
- Examine respiratory system – listen for signs of heart failure.
- Request chest x-ray – look for signs of heart failure.

Circulation

- Obtain ECG – adverse sign is heart rate <40 beats/minute.
- Assess heart rate and rhythm.
- Record blood pressure – adverse sign is systolic BP <90 mmHg.
- Gain IV access.
- Obtain venous blood for U&E, FBC, cardiac enzymes or Troponin depending on local policies.
- If any adverse signs are present give atropine 500 mcg IV.
- Repeat dose every 3–5 minutes up to a maximum of 3 mg.
- Consider referral to cardiologist for pacing if there is a risk of asystole.

Disability

- Assess conscious level using AVPU.

Exposure

- Once the patient is stable a detailed, structured history and examination can be undertaken.

ASSESSMENT FOR RISK OF ASYSTOLE

Following administration of atropine it is necessary to assess a patient's risk of developing asystole. If the patient has any of the following features, prompt referral for consideration of pacing is required:

- recent asystole
- Mobitz II atrioventricular (AV) block
- complete AV block (3rd degree heart block)
- ventricular standstill of >3 seconds

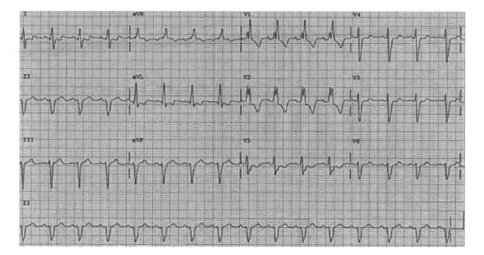

Figure 6.6. Mobitz Type II.

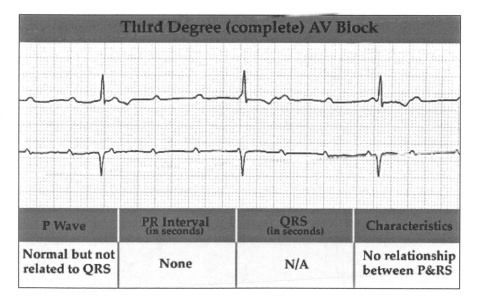

Figure 6.7. Complete AV block. Reproduced with kind permission of Frank Yanowitz.

TACHYCARDIA

DEFINITION

Tachycardia is defined as a heart rate of >100 beats per minute. A heart rate of 100 beats per minute is frequently a normal response to, for example, exercise or infection. It is usually when a heart rate exceeds 150 beats per minute that a patient becomes symptomatic and requires prompt treatment.

ADVERSE SIGNS

Adverse features of a tachycardia are:

- systolic BP <90 mmHg
- heart rate >150 beats/minute
- chest pain
- heart failure
- drowsiness
- confusion

ASSESSMENT

As always, follow an ABCDE approach to assessment.

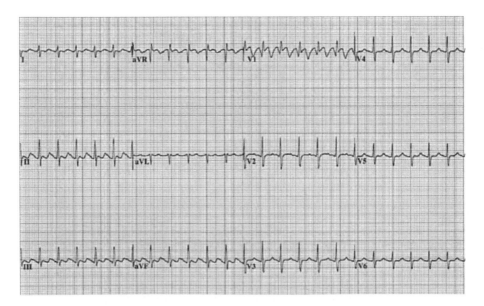

Figure 6.8. Narrow complex tachycardia.

Airway

- Assess and maintain airway.
- Utilise head tilt, chin lift if necessary.
- Use airway adjuncts if required.
- Consider urgent referral to anaesthetist for intubation if unable to protect airway.

Breathing

- Assess oxygen saturations using pulse oximeter – aim to maintain saturations at >92%.
- Give high flow oxygen via non re-breath mask.
- Assess respiratory rate.
- Examine respiratory system – listen for signs of heart failure.
- Request chest x-ray – look for signs of heart failure.

Circulation

- Obtain ECG – adverse sign is heart rate >150 beats/minute.
- Assess heart rate and rhythm – is this broad or narrow complex tachycardia?
- Record blood pressure – adverse sign is systolic BP <90 mmHg.
- Gain IV access.
- Obtain venous blood for U&E, FBC, cardiac enzymes or Troponin depending on local policies.

If Patient Unstable

- Summon medical assistance immediately.
- Patient requires DC cardioversion by an expert.
- Following three attempts at cardioversion give amiodarone 300 mg IV over 10–20 minutes.
- Repeat attempts at cardioversion can then be made.
- Follow this with an infusion of amiodarone 900 mg over 24 hours.

If the patient is stable it is vital to determine if this is a broad or narrow complex tachycardia as this determines your course of action.

If Patient Stable and Broad Complex Tachycardia

- Summon medical assistance.
- Is the rhythm regular or irregular?

If Regular

- If this is ventricular tachycardia (VT) – give amiodarone 300 mg IV over 10–20 minutes followed by 900 mg IV over 24 hours.

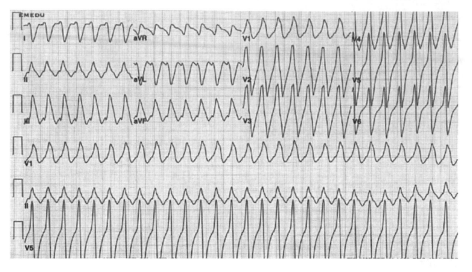

Figure 6.9. Broad complex tachycardia (VT).

- If previously know supra-ventricular tachycardia (SVT) with bundle branch block – give adenosine 6 mg rapid IV bolus followed by 12 mg and further 12 mg if unsuccessful.

If Irregular

- If this is atrial fibrillation (AF) see AF guideline in next section.
- If this is pre-excited AF – give amiodarone 300 mg IV over 10–20 minutes followed by 900 mg IV over 24 hours.
- If this is torsade de pointes – give magnesium 2 g IV over 10 minutes.

If Patient Stable and Narrow Complex Tachycardia

- Summon medical assistance.
- Is the rhythm regular or irregular?

If Regular

- Use vagal manoeuvres – before using carotid sinus massage, listen for carotid bruit. If bruit present do not use this method of vagal manoeuvre.
- Give adenosine 6 mg by rapid IV bolus.
- If unsuccessful, give 12 mg rapid IV bolus.
- If unsuccessful, give further 12 mg IV.
- Monitor ECG continuously during this time.

- Warn the patient that they may develop some chest pain and feel very 'strange' during administration.
- If normal sinus rhythm returns – record ECG.
- If this recurs adenosine can be given again but referral to a cardiologist should be made.

If Irregular

- This is likely to be AF – follow guideline in next section.

Do not forget to complete your assessment.

Disability

- Assess conscious level using AVPU.

Exposure

- Once the patient is stable a detailed, structured history and examination can be undertaken.

ATRIAL FIBRILLATION (AF)

DEFINITION

Atrial fibrillation is defined as chaotic atrial activity, rendering the atrium mechanically ineffective. The AV node conducts a proportion of the atrial impulses, resulting in an irregular ventricular response. It is characterised by an irregularly irregular pulse. AF may be paroxysmal in nature or continuous.

Atrial fibrillation is the commonest sustained cardiac arrhythmia. If it is left untreated it carries a significant risk of stroke and other morbidities. Hence in June 2006 NICE issued guidance on the management of AF.

What follows reflects the management suggested by NICE. Further information on this guidance can be found at www.nice.org.uk

SYMPTOMS AND SIGNS

There are many people in the community with AF in whom it is not a major medical problem as it is well controlled with medication. Within the MAU setting AF becomes a clinical problem usually when the rate is fast or AF is of new onset.

Palpitations are often the patient's main physical complaint. However patients with AF may present with the following:

- shortness of breath
- palpitations

- syncope
- dizziness
- chest pain
- TIA
- CVA

ASSESSMENT

As always, follow an ABCDE approach to assessment.

Airway

- Assess and maintain airway.
- Utilise head tilt, chin lift if necessary.
- Use airway adjuncts if required.
- Consider urgent referral to anaesthetist for intubation if unable to protect airway.

Breathing

- Assess oxygen saturations using pulse oximeter – aim to maintain saturations at >92%.
- Give high-flow oxygen via non re-breath mask.
- Assess respiratory rate.
- Examine respiratory system – listen for signs of heart failure.
- Request chest x-ray – look for signs of heart failure.

Circulation

- Obtain ECG.
- Assess heart rate and rhythm.
- Record blood pressure.
- Gain IV access.
- Obtain venous blood for U&E, FBC, cardiac enzymes or Troponin, depending on local policies.
- Commence heparin – this may be LMWH or IV heparin, depending on local policy.
- If the patient is haemodynamically unstable, which may be life-threatening – refer to cardiologist immediately as emergency cardioversion should be considered.
- If the patient is clinically unstable but this is not life-threatening – refer to cardiology as cardioversion is recommended.
- If cardioversion is to be delayed administer amiodarone 300 mg IV.
- If heart rate remains unstable, IV treatment with one of the following should be considered:

- beta blocker
- rate limiting calcium antagonists
- amiodarone.

Disability

- Assess using AVPU.
- Assess stroke risk:

Patients at High Risk of Stroke

- previous TIA/CVA or thromboembolic event
- age ≥75 with
  - hypertension
  - diabetes
  - vascular disease
- clinical evidence of:
  - valve disease
  - heart failure
  - impaired LV function on echo

Patients at Moderate Risk of Stroke

- age ≥65 with no risk factors
- age <75 with
  - hypertension
  - diabetes
  - vascular disease

Patients at Low Risk of Stroke

- age 65 with no moderate or high risk factors

For Patients in the High Risk Group

- if no contraindications to warfarin anticoagulate, aim for a target INR of 2.5
- if there are contraindications to warfarin, commence aspirin 75–300 mg once daily

For Patients in the Moderate Risk Group

- consider anticoagulation with warfarin on an individual basis balancing the risks and benefits
- if warfarin is not used, commence aspirin 75–300 mg once daily

For Patients in the Low Risk Group

- commence aspirin 75–300 mg once daily
- the GP should be asked to reassess risk on an individual basis

Exposure

- If you have not already done so, undertake a detailed history and clinical examination.
- If the cause of AF has not been established, look for any obvious causes now.

CARDIAC FAILURE

DEFINITION

Cardiac failure occurs when the heart is unable to maintain sufficient cardiac output to meet demand despite normal venous pressures. Cardiac failure can be of acute onset or a chronic problem. This section outlines the management of acute cardiac failure, a common presenting problem in MAU.

SIGNS AND SYMPTOMS

Patients presenting with cardiac failure present with the following:

- dyspnoea
- orthopnoea
- paroxysmal nocturnal dyspnoea (PND)
- oedema of ankles, lower limbs and in severe cases buttocks
- fatigue
- cough and frothy or pink sputum
- tachycardia

ASSESSMENT

As always, follow an ABCDE approach to assessment.

Airway

- Assess and maintain airway.
- Utilise head tilt, chin lift if necessary.
- Use airway adjuncts if required.
- Consider urgent referral to anaesthetist for intubation if unable to protect airway.

Breathing

- Sit patient up to assist breathing.
- Assess oxygen saturations using pulse oximeter – aim to maintain saturations at >92%.
- Obtain arterial blood gas if hypoxic to assess PaO_2 and $PaCO_2$.
- Give high-flow oxygen via non re-breath mask unless known COPD – in which case give 24% until blood gases obtained.
- Consider assisting breathing with bag-valve-mask ventilation.
- Assess respiratory rate.
- Examine respiratory system.
- Listen for:
  - crackles
  - decreased air entry
  - wheeze.
- Request chest x-ray – look for:
  - cardiomegaly
  - pleural effusions
  - fluid in the horizontal interlobar fissure
  - upper lobe venous engorgement.

Circulation

- Assess heart rate and rhythm – a third or fourth heart sound may be heard.
- Record blood pressure.
- Obtain ECG – may give indication of the underlying cause such as ischaemia or arrhythmia
- Gain IV access.
- Obtain venous blood for U&E, FBC, LFT's, cardiac enzymes or Troponin depending on local policy.
- Insert urinary catheter and monitor urine output hourly.
- Maintain strict fluid balance chart.
- Give furosemide 40 mg by slow IV injection (rate of 4 mg/minute).
- Medical assistance should be summoned.
- Diamorphine 5 mg by slow IV injection is recommended. If the patient is frail elderly give 2.5 mg IV.
- If systolic BP is >100 mmHg consider giving IV GTN – dilute 50 mg to a solution of 50 mls with 0.9% sodium chloride or 5% glucose. Commence infusion at rate of 20 mcg/minute and titrate according to BP response in 20 mcg increments at 15–30 minute intervals, to a maximum of 200 mcg/minute.
- GTN should be titrated to keep BP ≥90/60 mmHg.
- If systolic BP <100 mmHg consider IV dobutamine – dilute 250 mg to solution of 50 mls with 0.9% sodium chloride or 5% glucose for infusion via syringe. Weigh patient. Titrate infusion at a rate of 2.5–10 mcg/kg according to BP, heart rate and urine output.

- Once the patient is stable and out of the acute phase an ACE inhibitor should be considered along with maintenance diuretic therapy.
- Once stable, weigh daily to assess response to treatment.

Disability

- Assess conscious level using AVPU.

Exposure

- Once the patient is stable a detailed, structured history and examination can be undertaken.

DEEP VEIN THROMBOSIS (DVT)

DVT is often asymptomatic but left untreated can cause major problems, including PE and cardiac arrest.

DEFINITION

DVT is the formation of a thrombus in any vein. However, the most common sites for formation are the pelvis and leg.

SIGNS AND SYMPTOMS

Patients are often asymptomatic; frequently first presentation is with the signs and symptoms of a PE. Those that do present with symptoms of a DVT often complain of:

- swelling of the calf or leg
- their leg being warm to touch
- superficial veins being distended
- pain
- their leg feeling stiff
- pitting oedema
- erythema
- mild pyrexia

RISK FACTORS

It is important to assess the risks of DVT:

- recent surgery
- recent trauma
- immobility for any reason
- malignancy

- patients taking the oral contraceptive pill
- patients on hormone replacement therapy
- late pregnancy
- obesity
- patients taking Selective Estregen Receptor Modulator therapy (SERM)
- hyperviscosity syndromes
- pureperium
- nephrotic syndrome
- defective fibrinolysis
- antithrombin III deficiency
- protein C and protein S deficiency
- lupus anticoagulant

ASSESSMENT

As always, follow an ABCDE approach to assessment.

Airway

- Assess and maintain airway.

Breathing

- Assess oxygen saturations using pulse oximeter – aim to maintain saturations at > 92%.
- If patient is hypoxic give high-flow oxygen and consider PE as a diagnosis and follow treatment guidelines in Chapter 5.
- Assess respiratory rate.
- Examine respiratory system.

Circulation

- Assess heart rate and rhythm.
- Record blood pressure.
- Consider the need for IV access.
- Obtain venous blood for FBC, D-dimer and INR.
- Examine lower limbs for signs of swelling, pitting oedema, engorged superficial veins and evidence of cellulitis.
- Perform abdominal examination as a pelvic mass is a common cause of DVT.
- Measure both calves 10 cm below the tibial tuberosity.
- Weigh patient and give appropriate dose of low molecular weight heparin.
- Assess pre-test probability according to Wells score (Wells et al. 1997).
- Request Doppler ultrasound as indicted by Wells score.

Clinical Features
Score 1 point for each of the following features. In patients with symptoms in both legs use the more symptomatic leg.

- Active cancer (treatment within 6 months, ongoing or palliative).
- Paralysis, paresis or recent plaster immobilisation of legs.
- Bedridden for >3 days or major surgery under GA within last 12 weeks.
- Localised tenderness along distribution of deep venous system.
- Entire leg swollen.
- Calf circumference 3 cm greater than asymptomatic leg (measured 10 cm below tibial tuberosity).
- Pitting oedema (confined to symptomatic leg).
- Collateral superficial veins (non-varicose).
- Previously documented DVT.

Deduct 2 points if an alternative diagnosis is at least as likely as DVT.

Score	Pre-test probability
≥3	75% (high)
1–2	17% (moderate)
≤ 0	3% (low)

Figure 6.10. Pre-test clinical scoring for DVT. *Source:* PS Wells et al. (1997) Pre-test clinical scoring for DVT. Reproduced with kind permission of Elsevier.

- If Doppler positive anticoagulate in accordance with Fennerty regime (see PE management. Chapter 5. Figure 5.4).
- If Doppler negative, manage according to pre-test probability:
  - ➤ if pre-test probability low/moderate and Doppler negative – DVT excluded
  - ➤ if pre-test probability high, Doppler negative and D-dimer negative – DVT excluded
  - ➤ if pre-test probability high, Doppler negative and Ddimer positive – do not anticoagulate but repeat the Doppler scan in 4–7 days.

Disability

- Assess conscious level using AVPU.

Exposure

- Once the patient is stable, a detailed, structured history and examination can be undertaken.

AORTIC DISSECTION

DEFINITION

An aneurysm is an increase in the normal diameter of a blood vessel by 50%. Aneurysms are usually caused by atheroma and are frequently an incidental finding on examination. They may be felt as a pulsatile mass on abdominal examination or seen as calcification on a plain x-ray.

Aortic dissection refers to the rupture of this vessel. A vessel rupture is often a catastrophic event. Immediate referral to cardiology and cardiothoracic surgeons is paramount if chances of survival are to be optimised. Mortality is 1% per hour (Erbel et al. 2001).

SYMPTOMS AND SIGNS

Patients with aortic dissection present with:

- severe pain in the chest of sudden onset
- pain which patients often describe as a tearing pain
- pain may radiate to the back, iliac fossae and groins
- paraplegia as a result of tearing of the anterior spinal artery
- shortness of breath
- collapse with loss of consciousness
- unequal arm pulses and blood pressure
- evidence of limb and/or abdominal ischaemia

ASSESSMENT

Prompt recognition and assessment is vital. As always, follow an ABCDE approach to assessment.

Airway

- Assess and maintain airway.
- Utilise head tilt, chin lift if necessary.
- Use airway adjuncts if required.
- Consider urgent referral to anaesthetist for intubation if unable to protect airway.
- A patient with aortic dissection is likely to need ITU admission – summon medical help now.

Breathing

- Assess oxygen saturations using pulse oximeter – aim to maintain saturations at >92%.
- Give high-flow oxygen via non re-breath mask.
- Consider assisting breathing with bag-valve-mask ventilation.
- Assess respiratory rate.
- Examine respiratory system.
- Request chest x-ray.

Circulation

- Assess heart rate and rhythm.
- Place patient on a cardiac monitor.
- Record blood pressure in both arms.
- Obtain an ECG – evidence of ischaemia is likely and there may also be changes consistent with MI.
- Gain IV access – two large bore cannulae.
- Obtain venous blood for U&E, FBC, Creatinine Kinase (CK) Troponin and myoglobin if available, D-dimer and LDH.
- Give the patient IV analgesia – morphine 5 mg initially and titrate upwards as tolerated.
- Refer urgently to cardiology and cardiothoracic surgeons for intervention.
- If the patient is hypertensive, BP can be reduced with IV beta blockers. This should only be done with expert advice from cardiology – agents that can be used are propanolol, metoprolol, esmolol and labetolol.
- If hypertension is severe IV sodium nitroprusside can be given but only under supervision of cardiology and intensivists.
- Discuss with cardiology the urgent need for an echo.
- A CT or MRI scan may be indicated under the guidance of cardiology.

Disability

- Assess conscious level using AVPU.
- A deteriorating level of consciousness is indication for referral to ITU.
- Patients with aortic dissection are at high risk of cardiac arrest.

Exposure

- If the patient stabilises, a full detailed history and clinical examination may be undertaken. However the patient may be transferred to theatre or ITU before this can be done.

CARDIAC TAMPONADE

DEFINITION

Cardiac tamponade is a medical emergency. A large amount of fluid accumulates in the pericardium. As a result there is pressure around the heart which prevents proper filling of the heart cavities. Instead of reducing the filling of both ventricles equally, the septum of the heart bends into either the left or right ventricle. The result is low stroke volume and shock.

SYMPTOMS AND SIGNS

Patients with cardiac tamponade may present with:

- shortness of breath
- tachycardia
- sweating
- appearance of paleness
- the patient may have a decreased level of consciousness
- possible clinical signs of shock
- poor urine output
- signs of a raised JVP on examination
- pulsus paradoxus
- soft heart sounds
- a history of recent chest trauma or myocardial infarction

LIFE-THREATENING FEATURES

- tachycardia >100 beats per minute
- systolic BP <100 mmHg
- hypotension during inspiration
- echo evidence of right ventricular diastolic collapse
- large pleural effusion on chest x-ray

ASSESSMENT

Prompt recognition and assessment is vital. As always, follow an ABCDE approach to assessment.

Airway

- Assess and maintain airway.
- Utilise head tilt, chin lift if necessary.
- Use airway adjuncts if required.
- Consider urgent referral to anaesthetist for intubation if unable to protect airway.
- Get expert help now – you are going to need it.

Breathing

- Assess oxygen saturations using pulse oximeter – aim to maintain saturations at >92%.
- Give high-flow oxygen via non re-breath mask.
- Consider assisting breathing with bag-valve-mask ventilation.
- Assess respiratory rate.

- Examine respiratory system.
- Request chest x-ray – look for signs of pleural effusion.

Circulation

- Assess heart rate and rhythm.
- Place patient on a cardiac monitor.
- Obtain an ECG – look for signs of right heart strain and possible MI.
- Gain IV access – two large bore cannulae.
- Obtain venous blood for U&E, FBC, cross match, INR.
- Give the patient IV analgesia – morphine 5 mg initially and titrate upwards as tolerated.
- Refer urgently to cardiology.
- Discuss with cardiology the urgent need for an echo.
- Liaise with cardiology re pericardial aspiration.

Disability

- Assess conscious level using AVPU.
- A deteriorating level of consciousness is indication for referral to ITU.
- Patients with cardiac tamponade are at high risk of cardiac arrest.

Exposure

- If the patient stabilises a full detailed history and clinical examination may be undertaken. However the patient may be transferred to ITU before this can be done.

REFERENCES

Erbel R, Alfonso F, Boileau C, Dirsch O, Eber B, Haverich A et al. (2001) Diagnosis and management of aortic dissection. *European Heart Journal* Sep 22(18): 1642–81.

Fennerty A, Dolben J and Thomas P (1984) Flexible induction dose regimen for warfarin and predictive maintenance dose. *British Medical Journal* 288: 1268–70.

Malmberg K, Ryden L, Efendic S, Herlitz, J, Nicol P, Waldenstrom A et al. (1995) Randomised trial of insulin-glucose infusion followed by subcutaneous insulin treatment in diabetic patients with acute myocardial infarction (DIGAMI study) effects on mortality at 1 year. *Journal of American College of Cardiology* 26: 57–65.

National Institute for Clinical Excellence (2006) *Atrial Fibrillation: The Management of Atrial Fibrillation.* Clinical Guideline 36. London: NICE.

National Service Framework (2000) *Coronary Heart Disease: National Service Framework for Coronary Heart Disease – Modern Standards and Service Model.* London: Department of Health.

Resuscitation Council UK (2005) *Advanced Life Support Guidelines*. London: Resuscitation Council UK.

Tsang TS, Oh JK and Seward JB (1999) Diagnosis and management of cardiac tamponade in the era of echocardiography. *Clinical Cardiology* 22(7): 446–52.

Wells PS, Anderson DR, Bormains J, Guy F, Mitchell M, Gray L et al. (1997) Value of assessment of pre-test probability of deep vein thrombosis in clinical management. *Lancet* 350: 1795–8.

7 Gatrointestinal Conditions

Chronic peptic ulceration is the most common cause of gastrointestinal haemorrhage. The mortality rate is 5–10%. Therefore prompt recognition and assessment is important.

UPPER GASTROINTESTINAL BLEEDING (GI BLEED)

DEFINITION

- Haematemesis is the vomiting of blood.
- Malaena is the passage of black tarry stools.

Common causes of GI bleed are:

- duodenal/gastric ulceration
- gastritis/gastric crosions
- Mallory-Weiss tear
- duodenitis
- oesophagitis
- oesophageal varices
- malignancy
- drug induced – non-steroidals and anticoagulants

SYMPTOMS AND SIGNS

Patients with a GI bleed may present with the following:

- coffee ground vomiting
- haematemesis
- malaena
- postural hypotension
- abdominal pain
- signs of anaemia:
  - lcthargy
  - shortness of breath

- signs of shock:
  - ➤ tachycardia
  - ➤ hypotension
  - ➤ cold and clammy
- signs of liver disease

Patients with signs of shock require immediate medical assistance and fluid resuscitation.

LIFE-THREATENING FEATURES

It is essential to identify those patients at high risk of death. If one or more of the following are present, the patient is at high risk of death and requires urgent medical intervention.

- tachycardia >100 beats per minute
- systolic BP <100 mmHg
- postural hypotension – a fall of ≥ 10 mmHg
- severe liver, cardiovascular, respiratory or renal disease
- disseminated malignancy
- re-bleeding after admission
- haemoglobin <10 g/dl

ASSESSMENT

As always, follow an ABCDE approach to assessment.

Airway

- Assess and maintain airway.
- Utilise head tilt, chin lift if necessary.
- Use airway adjuncts if required.
- Consider urgent referral to anaesthetist for intubation if unable to protect airway.

Breathing

- Assess oxygen saturations using pulse oximeter – aim to maintain saturations at >92%.
- Give high flow oxygen via non re-breath mask.
- Obtain arterial blood gases if hypoxia persists.
- Assess respiratory rate.
- Examine respiratory system.
- Request chest x-ray.

Circulation

- Assess heart rate and rhythm.
- Record blood pressure.
- Gain IV access – two large-bore cannulae.
- Give IV fluids – sodium chloride 0.9% over 30 mins–1 hour.
- If hypotensive give Gelofusine 500 mls stat and continue until systolic BP > 100 mmHg.
- Obtain venous blood for cross match, U&E, FBC, LFTs and INR.
- If the patient is in extremis give O negative blood, otherwise await cross-matched blood.
- Insert urinary catheter and monitor output hourly.
- Refer for urgent gastroscopy as per local policy.
- Commence IV proton pump inhibitor (PPI) – omeprazole 80 mg IV as a stat dose followed by an infusion at a rate of 8 mg an hour for 72 hours.

Disability

- Assess conscious level using AVPU.

Exposure

- Once the patient is stable a detailed, structured history and examination can be undertaken.

VARICEAL BLEEDING

Oesophageal varices pose a life-threatening event when they bleed. The patient will require immediate resuscitation and intervention. Medical assistance must be summoned immediately and the help of a gastroenterologist for possible insertion of a Sengstaken-Blakemore tube is recommended.

Patients present with signs of shock and massive haematemesis.

ASSESSMENT

As always, follow an ABCDE approach to assessment.

Airway

- Assess and maintain airway.
- Utilise head tilt, chin lift if necessary.
- Use airway adjuncts if required.
- Consider urgent referral to anaesthetist for intubation if unable to protect airway.

Breathing

- Assess oxygen saturations using pulse oximeter – aim to maintain saturations at >92%.
- Give high-flow oxygen via non re-breath mask.
- Obtain arterial blood gases if hypoxia persists.
- Assess respiratory rate.
- Full respiratory examination can wait until the patient is stable.

Circulation

- Assess heart rate and rhythm.
- Record blood pressure.
- Assess jugular venous pressure (JVP).
- Gain IV access – two large-bore cannulae.
- Give IV fluids – sodium chloride 0.9% over 30 mins–1 hour.
- If hypotensive, give Gelofusine 500 mls stat and continue until systolic BP >100 mmHg.
- Obtain venous blood for cross match, U&E, FBC, LFTs and INR.
- If the patient is in extremis give O negative blood, otherwise await cross-matched blood.
- Insert urinary catheter and monitor output hourly.
- Refer for urgent gastroscopy.
- Commence octreotide IV – dilute 500 mcg in 50 mls of sodium chloride 0.9% and infuse at rate of 5 ml/hour (50 mcg/hr).
- If bleeding continues gain urgent expert help from a gastroenterologist for insertion of a Sengstaken-Blakemore tube.
- Consider the need for a central venous pressure line (CVP).
- Obtain blood cultures.
- Commence antibiotics – co-amoxiclav 375 mg orally or 1.2 g IV 8 hourly.

Disability

- Assess conscious level using AVPU.
- Commence treatment to avoid hepatic encephalopathy (see next section). A large variceal bleed is the equivalent of a large protein meal and the risk of encephalopathy is high.

Exposure

- Once the patient is stable, a detailed, structured history and examination can be undertaken.
- 40% of patients who re-bleed will die.
- Observe for signs of re-bleed:

- ➢ rising pulse rate
- ➢ falling JVP
- ➢ decreasing hourly urine output
- ➢ haematemesis
- ➢ malaena
- ➢ fall in BP.
- If there is evidence of a re-bleed, summon urgent medical assistance.

ACUTE LIVER FAILURE WITH ENCEPHALOPATHY

Liver failure may occur as a result of an acute insult on the liver in a previously fit and healthy adult. More frequently it is a result of decompensation following chronic liver disease.

DEFINITION

Fulminant hepatic failure is defined as hepatic failure with encephalopathy developing in less than two weeks, in a patient with a previously healthy liver, or in patients with an acute exacerbation of chronic liver disease.

SIGNS AND SYMPTOMS

Patients with acute liver failure and encephalopathy may present with:

- malaise
- nausea and vomiting
- bruising
- petechiae
- jaundice
- altered conscious level
- ascites
- oedema
- flap – a coarse irregular tremor

LIFE-THREATENING FEATURES

- patient exhausted
- hypotension despite IV fluids
- inotrope dependence
- hypoglycaemia
- metabolic acidosis
- pulmonary oedema
- oliguria or anuria

- spontaneous bruising or bleeding
- cerebral oedema
- bradycardia
- papilloedema

ASSESSMENT

Liver failure should be considered in all patients with abnormal liver function and an altered level of consciousness.

As always, follow an ABCDE approach to assessment.

Airway

- Assess and maintain airway.
- Utilise head tilt, chin lift if necessary.
- Use airway adjuncts if required.
- Consider urgent referral to anaesthetist for intubation if unable to protect airway.

Breathing

- Assess oxygen saturations using pulse oximeter – aim to maintain saturations at >92%.
- Give high-flow oxygen via non re-breath mask.
- Obtain arterial blood gases to assess pH, PaO_2 and $PaCO_2$.
- Assess respiratory rate.
- Examine respiratory system – look for signs of pulmonary oedema.
- Request chest x-ray – look for signs of pulmonary oedema.

Circulation

- Assess heart rate and rhythm.
- Record blood pressure.
- Obtain ECG.
- Assess jugular venous pressure (JVP).
- Gain IV access – two large-bore cannulae.
- Summon medical assistance.
- Give IV fluids if hypotensive – give Gelofusine 500 mls stat and continue until systolic BP >100 mmHg.
- Obtain venous blood for U&E, FBC, LFTs, INR, paracetamol levels, blood glucose, hepatitis A and B serology.
- Insert urinary catheter and monitor output hourly.
- Consider the need for a central venous pressure line (CVP) – summon medical assistance.

Grade	Symptoms and signs
1	Confused
	Altered mood or behaviour
2	Drowsy with inappropriate behaviour
3	Stupor with inarticulate speech. Rousable and can obey simple commands. Severe agitation, wailing and decerebrate posturing
4	Coma
	Unrousable

Figure 7.1. West Haven Criteria for Grading Encephalopathy. *Source:* HO Conn (1977) Quantifying the severity of hepatic encephalopathy. *American Journal of Digestive Disorders* 22: 541–50.

- Obtain blood cultures.
- Obtain urine for culture and sensitivity.
- If the patient is unable to take medication orally, insert naso-gastric tube.
- If the patient remains hypotensive, consider the need for inotropes – seek medical assistance now if you have not already done so.
- Commence prophylactic antibiotics – co-amoxiclav 1.2 g IV eight-hourly or ciprofloxacin 200 mg IV and metronidazole 500 mg IV 12 hourly. Check local antibiotic policy first. These can be amended once culture results are available.
- Correct hypoglycaemia – give glucose 5% IV.
- If there is evidence of bleeding or bruising and raised INR, give vitamin K 10 mg IV by slow infusion – dilute in 55 mls glucose 5%.
- If the patient is actively bleeding, consider administering fresh frozen plasma.

Disability

- Assess conscious level using AVPU.
- Assess grade of encephalopathy using West Haven Criteria (1977).
- Ensure lactulose is prescribed and administered.

Exposure

- Once the patient is stable a detailed, structured history and examination can be undertaken.
- Do not forget to ensure fundoscopy is performed to assess papilloedema.

ACUTE ULCERATIVE COLITIS AND CROHN'S DISEASE

Acute exacerbations of ulcerative colitis (UC) and Crohn's disease can be life-threatening and require prompt assessment and treatment.

DEFINITION

Ulcerative colitis is defined as an inflammatory disorder of the colonic mucosa. It is characterised by relapses and remissions. UC usually affects just the colon but can equally involve all or part of the colon (Carter et al. 2004).

Crohn's disease is defined as a chronic inflammatory disease characterised by transmural granulomatous inflammation. It can affect any part of the gut but is more usually seen in the terminal ileum and proximal colon (Kumar and Clarke 2003).

SIGNS AND SYMPTOMS

The signs and symptoms of UC and Crohn's are very similar and initial management in the acute phase is identical. For this reason the two conditions will be dealt with together.

Patients with UC and Crohn's may present with:

- abdominal pain
- diarrhoea
- blood in stool
- fever
- malaise
- weight loss
- signs of anaemia
- tachycardia
- signs of dehydration

LIFE-THREATENING FEATURES

If patients exhibit any of the following life-threatening features, summon medical assistance and refer to the surgeons for an urgent opinion.

- signs of severe sepsis
- septic shock
- toxic dilatation of the colon
- severe disturbance of U&E
- haemorrhage
- multi-organ failure

ASSESSMENT

As always, use an ABCDE approach to assessment.

Airway

- Assess and maintain airway.
- Utilise head tilt, chin lift if necessary.

- Use airway adjuncts if required.
- Consider urgent referral to anaesthetist for intubation if unable to protect airway.

Breathing

- Assess oxygen saturations using pulse oximeter – aim to maintain saturations at >92%.
- Give high-flow oxygen via non re-breath mask if hypoxic.
- Obtain arterial blood gases to assess pH, PaO_2 and $PaCO_2$.
- Assess respiratory rate.
- Examine respiratory system.
- Request erect chest x-ray – look for gas under the diaphragm.

Circulation

- Assess heart rate and rhythm.
- Record blood pressure.
- Obtain ECG.
- Gain IV access – two large-bore cannulae.
- Summon medical assistance.
- Give IV fluids – if hypotensive give Gelofusine 500 mls stat and continue until systolic BP >100 mmHg.
- If no hypotension but evidence of dehydration on U&E, administer sodium chloride 0.9% over two hours or dextrose saline.
- Obtain venous blood for U&E, FBC, LFTs, blood glucose and cross match.
- Obtain blood cultures.
- Obtain urine for culture and sensitivity.
- Obtain stool for culture.
- If Hb <8 g/dL transfuse 4 units of blood.
- Commence hydrocortisone 200 mg IV eight-hourly.
- Commence metronidazole 500 mg IV eight-hourly.

Disability

- Assess conscious level using AVPU.

Exposure

- Once the patient is stable a detailed, structured history and examination can be undertaken. This should include a thorough abdominal examination.
- Request abdominal x-ray – look for dilated bowel loops.
- Refer to a gastroenterologist for further investigation (colonoscopy and/or barium enema) once the acute phase is over.

REFERENCES

Carter MJ, Lobo AJ and Travis SP (2004) Guidelines for the management of inflammatory bowel disease in adults. *Gut* 53. Suppl. V: v1–v16.

Conn HO (1977) Quantifying the severity of hepatic encephalopathy. *American Journal of Digestive Disorders* 22: 541–50.

Kumar P and Clark M (2003) *Clinical Medicine*, 3rd edn. London: Saunders.

Longmore M, Wilkinson I and Török E (2001) *Oxford Handbook of Clinical Medicine*, 5th edn. Oxford: Oxford University Press.

8 Metabolic Conditions

Metabolic emergencies, although not as common as some of the other conditions already covered, are frequently seen in the medical assessment unit. They all require prompt assessment, diagnosis and treatment. This chapter covers the metabolic conditions most commonly seen in MAU.

DIABETIC KETOACIDOSIS (DKA)

DEFINITION

Diabetic ketoacidosis results from grossly deficient insulin availability, causing a transition from glucose to lipid oxidation and metabolism. In type 1 diabetes DKA is commonly caused by a lapse in insulin treatment or by an acute infection, trauma, or infarction that makes usual insulin treatment inadequate. Patients with type 2 diabetes rarely suffer from DKA.

SYMPTOMS AND SIGNS

Patients with DKA present with the following:

- thirst
- polyuria
- flushed appearance
- Kussmaul breathing (sighing respirations)
- smell of ketones on the breath
- dehydration
- drowsiness

LIFE-THREATENING FEATURES

- coma
- severe acidosis – pH <6.8
- severe hypotension unresponsive to IV fluids

ASSESSMENT

As always, follow an ABCDE approach.

Airway

- Assess and maintain airway.
- Utilise head tilt, chin lift if necessary.
- Use airway adjuncts if required.
- Consider urgent referral to anaesthetist for intubation if unable to protect airway.

Breathing

- Assess oxygen saturations using pulse oximeter – aim to maintain saturations at >92%.
- Give high-flow oxygen via non re-breath mask.
- Assess respiratory rate.
- Examine respiratory system.
- Request chest x-ray – looking for signs of infection.

Circulation

- Summon medical help.
- Assess heart rate and rhythm.
- Record blood pressure – hypotension is a poor prognostic sign.
- Gain IV access.
- Obtain venous blood for U&E, FBC and glucose.
- Obtain arterial blood gases to assess severity of acidosis.
- Monitor blood glucose using capillary sample.
- Obtain an ECG.
- Insert urinary catheter and monitor output hourly if patient is unconscious or does not pass urine within three hours of starting IV fluids.
- Record patient's temperature.
- Obtain a MSU prior to starting antibiotics.
- If pyrexial obtain blood cultures and start a broad spectrum antibiotic in accordance with local policies (co-amoxiclav or erythromycin are suggestions).
- Test urine for ketones.
- Give IV fluids starting with 0.9% sodium chloride over 30 minutes.
- Subsequent IV fluid should be given over one hour, followed by 1 litre over two hours and then 1 litre over four hours.
- Potassium chloride should be infused in the IV fluid if serum potassium levels are <5.5 mmols.
- If potassium is being infused, monitor heart rate and rhythm.
- Commence an insulin infusion.
- Soluble insulin at a strength of 1 unit per ml in 0.9% sodium chloride via syringe pump should be used.
- Commence infusion at a rate of 6 units an hour.
- Monitor capillary blood glucose (BM) hourly.
- Once blood glucose is <15 mmols/l reduce insulin infusion to 3 units an hour and change IV fluid to 5% glucose.

- If serum potassium level remains <5.5, ensure 40 mmols potassium continues in subsequent bags of IV fluid.
- Monitor serum potassium every time IV fluid is changed.
- If blood glucose is <6 mmols/l reduce infusion to 1 unit an hour.
- Repeat arterial blood gases after initial IV insulin and fluid therapy.
- If patient remains acidotic and dehydrated, give IV 0.9% sodium chloride in conjunction with the IV glucose over eight hours.
- Do not give sodium bicarbonate.
- Sodium bicarbonate may be considered if pH <6.8 but should only be given by a specialist such as an ITU consultant. If a patient is this acidotic, they need ITU help.

Disability

- Assess level of consciousness using AVPU.
- Coma is an indication for referral to ITU.
- Observe for deterioration in level of consciousness. This may signify cerebral oedema requiring referral to ITU.

Exposure

- Once the patient is stable, a complete history and physical assessment can be undertaken.
- If no obvious cause of DKA has been found as yet, now is the time to search for a cause.

HYPEROSMOLAR NON-KETOTIC STATE (HONK)

DEFINITION

HONK is a clinical emergency in patients with type 2 diabetes. Patients develop severe hyperglycaemia without ketosis.

The clinical picture is usually one of insidious onset unlike the acute presentation of DKA. Mortality is 30–35% and increases with age, medical co-morbidity, severity of metabolic derangement and the degree of impairment of consciousness.

SYMPTOMS AND SIGNS

Patients with HONK present with very similar signs and symptoms as those with DKA.

- thirst
- polyuria
- flushed appearance
- Kussmaul breathing (sighing respirations)

- smell of ketones on the breath
- dehydration
- drowsiness
- seizures may be present

ASSESSMENT

The assessment and treatment of patients with HONK is the same as that for DKA with the exception that a lower dose of insulin is used. As always, follow an ABCDE approach.

Airway

- Assess and maintain airway.
- Utilise head tilt, chin lift if necessary.
- Use airway adjuncts if required.
- Consider urgent referral to anaesthetist for intubation if unable to protect airway.

Breathing

- Assess oxygen saturations using pulse oximeter – aim to maintain saturations at >92%.
- Give high-flow oxygen via non re-breath mask.
- Assess respiratory rate.
- Examine respiratory system.
- Request chest x-ray.

Circulation

- Summon medical help.
- Assess heart rate and rhythm.
- Record blood pressure.
- Gain IV access.
- Obtain venous blood for U&E, FBC and glucose.
- Obtain arterial blood gases to ensure absence of acidosis.
- Monitor blood glucose using capillary sample.
- Obtain an ECG.
- Insert urinary catheter and monitor output hourly if patient is unconscious or does not pass urine within three hours of starting IV fluids.
- Record patient's temperature.
- Obtain a MSU prior to starting antibiotics.
- If the patient is pyrexial, obtain blood cultures and start a broad spectrum antibiotic in accordance with local policies (co-amoxiclav or erythromycin are suggestions).
- Test urine for ketones.
- Give IV fluids starting with 0.9% sodium chloride over eight hours.

- Potassium chloride should be infused in the IV fluid if serum potassium levels are <5.5 mmols.
- If potassium is being infused monitor heart rate and rhythm.
- Commence an insulin infusion.
- Soluble insulin at a strength of 1 unit per ml in 0.9% sodium chloride via syringe pump.
- Commence infusion at a rate of 3 units an hour.
- Monitor capillary blood glucose (BM) hourly.
- If blood glucose does not fall after two hours double dose of insulin infusion to 6 units an hour.
- Once blood glucose is <15 mmols/l change IV fluid to 5% glucose.
- If serum potassium level remains <5.5 ensure 40 mmols potassium continues in subsequent bags of IV fluid.
- Monitor serum potassium every time IV fluid is changed.
- If blood glucose is <6 mmols/l reduce infusion to 1 unit an hour.

Disability

- Assess level of consciousness using AVPU.
- Coma is an indication for referral to ITU.
- Observe for deterioration in level of consciousness. This may signify cerebral oedema requiring referral to ITU.
- Monitor for seizures – patient will require monitoring in a high dependency area if seizures persist.

Exposure

- Once the patient is stable a complete history and physical assessment can be undertaken.

HYPOGLYCAEMIA

DEFINITION

Hypoglycaemia occurs when the serum glucose concentration falls below the normal 3.5–6.5 mmol/l.

Symptoms only usually occur when the serum glucose level falls below 2.5 mmol/l.

SYMPTOMS AND SIGNS

- cold and clammy skin
- confusion
- restlessness
- tachycardia

LIFE-THREATENING FEATURES

• coma

ASSESSMENT

As always, use an ABCDE approach.

Airway

• Assess and maintain airway.
• Utilise head tilt, chin lift if necessary.
• Use airway adjuncts if required.
• Consider urgent referral to anaesthetist for intubation if unable to protect airway.

Breathing

• Assess oxygen saturations using pulse oximeter – aim to maintain saturations at >92%.
• Give high-flow oxygen via non re-breath mask.
• Assess respiratory rate.
• A respiratory assessment and chest x-ray are not needed at this stage – consider if they are appropriate once the initial emergency has been dealt with.

Circulation

• Obtain capillary blood glucose (BM).
• Gain IV access.
• Obtain venous blood for U&E, LFTs and glucose.
• Record heart rate and blood pressure.
• A full cardiac assessment can wait until you have dealt with the acute emergency.

Disability

• Assess level of consciousness using AVPU.
• If the patient is able to protect their own airway and is semi-conscious:
  ➢ administer hypostop 23 g orally;
  ➢ this can be repeated after 10 minutes if necessary.
• If the patient is unconscious:
  ➢ administer 100 mls of 20% glucose IV over 15 minutes;
  ➢ if there is no improvement in blood glucose or the patient remains unconscious after 15 minutes, administer a further dose of 100 mls of 20% glucose IV;

➢ once the patient regains consciousness oral glucose and carbohydrate can be given.

Exposure

- A detailed history and physical assessment can be undertaken once the patient is stable.
- If the cause of the hypoglycaemia has not been found, now is the time to look for it.
- Consider the need for thyroid function tests (TFTs) and possibly short synacthen test.
- Patients who have a history of hypoglycaemia are only permitted to drive if they recognise the signs and symptoms of hypoglycaemia and have sufficient warning to allow them to take action. The DVLA state that if a patient is suffering from recurrent hypoglycaemic episodes they must cease driving until such time as they have gained satisfactory control of their blood sugars. DVLA only require a patient to notify them if they are suffering from recurrent hypoglycaemic episodes. Ensure your patient is aware of this and that it is documented in the medical notes.

HYPERGLYCAEMIA IN THE CRITICALLY ILL PATIENT

DEFINITION

Hyperglycaemia in the critically ill patient is defined as a blood glucose >12 mmol/l in any patient who is unwell for whatever reason. The patient does not have to be known previously to be diabetic (Mesotten and van den Berhe 2003).

The stress of critical illness is often accompanied by hyperglycaemia. It is considered to be due to the body's adaptive metabolic response to stress. The Diabetes and Insulin-Glucose infusion in Acute Myocardial Infarction (DIGAMI) study of 1995 by Malmberg et al. showed that in patients with diabetes, controlling blood glucose levels below 12 mmol/l for three months after MI improves long-term outcome (see Chapter 6, page 121 for further information on the DIGAMI regime). The Insulin in Intensive Care study by van den Berhe et al. (2001) looked at non-diabetic patients in critical care and showed that tight control of blood glucose improved outcome.

It is therefore important that all critically ill patients have assessment of blood glucose and, if found to be hyperglycaemic, receive appropriate insulin therapy.

SYMPTOMS AND SIGNS

The patient who is critically ill and has hyperglycaemia may not show any clinical signs that would lead the practitioner to suspect that they are hyperglycaemic. The potential for hyperglycaemia should be considered in the following circumstances:

- any patient who is acutely unwell for whatever reason
- patients who are known to have diabetes
- patients who are receiving corticosteroid treatment

ASSESSMENT

As always, use an ABCDE approach.

Airway

- Assess and maintain airway.
- Utilise head tilt, chin lift if necessary.
- Use airway adjuncts if required.
- Consider urgent referral to anaesthetist for intubation if unable to protect airway.

Breathing

- Assess oxygen saturations using pulse oximeter – aim to maintain saturations at >92%.
- Give high-flow oxygen via non re-breath mask.
- Assess respiratory rate.
- Examine respiratory system.
- Request chest x-ray.

Circulation

- Summon medical help if needed.
- Assess heart rate and rhythm.
- Record blood pressure.
- Gain IV access.
- Obtain venous blood for U&E, FBC and glucose.
- Obtain arterial blood gases to ensure absence of acidosis.
- If the patient has a metabolic acidosis treat as DKA and follow the DKA guideline.
- Monitor blood glucose using capillary sample.
- Obtain an ECG.
- Insert urinary catheter and monitor output hourly if patient is unconscious or does not pass urine within three hours of starting IV fluids.
- Record patient's temperature.
- Obtain a MSU prior to starting antibiotics.
- If the patient is pyrexial obtain blood cultures and consider starting a broad spectrum antibiotic in accordance with local policies (co-amoxiclav or erythromycin are suggestions).
- Test urine for ketones – if ketones present, consider the need to treat as DKA.
- Assess patient for signs of dehydration.

Stable Patients

If the patient is clinically stable, not dehydrated and able to eat but is persistently hyperglycaemic:

- If patient is usually on insulin – increase usual total daily insulin by 10–20%.
- If patient on oral diabetic medication – add a low dose of insulin, e.g. isophane 10 units.
- If not on any diabetic medication monitor blood glucose every four hours and consider treating as unstable if hyperglycaemia persists.

Unstable Patients

If the patient is clinically unstable, is dehydrated and has nausea and vomiting:

- Stop any usual diabetic medication.
- Give IV fluids starting with 0.9% sodium chloride – rate should be adjusted in accordance with degree of dehydration.
- Administer an insulin infusion – 50 units of soluble insulin (e.g. Actrapid) in 50 mls sodium chloride at a rate of 3 mls an hour.
- Monitor capillary blood glucose every two hours.
- If blood glucose >11 mmol/l after two hours, increase infusion by 1 unit/hour.
- If blood glucose 6–11 mmol/l after two hours, continue infusion at same rate.
- If blood glucose 3–5.9 mmol/l after two hours, reduce insulin infusion to 1 unit/hour and change IV fluid to 5% glucose.
- If blood glucose <3 mmmol/l after two hours, stop insulin infusion and administer 20% glucose (refer to hypoglycaemia guideline).

Disability

- Assess level of consciousness using AVPU.
- Coma is an indication for referral to ITU.
- Observe for deterioration in level of consciousness. This may signify cerebral oedema requiring referral to ITU.

Exposure

- Once the patient is stable, a complete history and physical assessment can be undertaken.
- Treat the underlying cause of hyperglycaemia.
- Patients will require conversion to their usual insulin regime or commencement of a basal bolus regime once they are clinically stable and able to eat and drink – this will be done on the ward and not in MAU.

HYPERCALCAEMIA

DEFINITION

Hypercalcaemia is defined as a serum calcium level above the normal (>2.6 mmol/l). It is categorised as mild, moderate or severe.

- mild = Ca^2 2.6–2.9 mmol/l
- moderate = Ca^2 3.0–3.4 mmol/l
- severe = Ca^2 >3.4 mmol/l

SYMPTOMS AND SIGNS

Patients do not usually have symptoms until calcium levels are >3.0 mmol/l. Presenting symptoms include:

- nausea and vomiting
- abdominal pain
- constipation
- polyuria
- polydipsia
- depression
- headache
- acute psychosis
- cognitive difficulties
- hypertension

LIFE-THREATENING SYMPTOMS

- altered level of consciousness
- ECG changes – prolonged QT and PR interval, a wide QRS complex and arrhythmias

ASSESSMENT

As always, use an ABCDE approach.

Airway

- Assess and maintain airway.
- Utilise head tilt, chin lift if necessary.
- Use airway adjuncts if required.
- Consider urgent referral to anaesthetist for intubation if unable to protect airway.

Breathing

- Assess oxygen saturations using pulse oximeter – aim to maintain saturations at >92%.
- Give high-flow oxygen via non re-breath mask.
- Assess respiratory rate.
- Examine respiratory system.
- Request chest x-ray.

Circulation

- Assess heart rate and rhythm.
- Record blood pressure.
- Gain IV access.
- Obtain venous blood for U&E, FBC, calcium, albumin, ESR, alkaline phosphatase, PTH and myeloma screen.
- Obtain an ECG.
- Assess severity of hypercalcaemia once corrected calcium is known.

Mild Hypercalcaemia

- Ensure adequate fluid intake.
- If on thiazide diuretics or vitamin A, D or calcium supplements ensure they are stopped.
- Acute inpatient management is not necessary but ensure that a referral to an endocrinologist is made for urgent follow up to determine the cause.

Moderate Hypercalcaemia – No Symptoms

- Rehydrate orally, aiming for 2–3 litres of water per day.
- If unable to achieve this orally give 0.9% sodium chloride IV.
- Patient will require a repeat calcium level in 48 hours. Ensure this is clearly documented in the management plan.

Moderate Hypercalcaemia – Symptoms Present

- Rehydrate with 0.9% sodium chloride IV.
- Patient will require 3–4 litres of IV fluid in the first 24 hours.
- Observe for signs of fluid overload.
- If evidence of fluid overload, give 20–40 mg furosemide IV at a maximum rate of 4 mg/min.
- If life-threatening features are present give calcitonin 4 units/kg IM every 12 hours for 24 hours.
- The patient will require a repeat calcium level 12 hours after starting treatment.
- Advice from an endocrinologist should be sought as soon as possible.

Severe Hypercalcaemia

- Rehydrate with 0.9% sodium chloride IV.
- Patient will require 3–4 litres of IV fluid in the first 24 hours.
- Observe for signs of fluid overload.
- If evidence of fluid overload give 20–40 mg furosemide IV at a maximum rate of 4 mg/min.
- If life-threatening features are present give calcitonin 4 units/kg IM every 12 hours for 24 hours.
- The patient will require a repeat calcium level 12 hours after starting treatment.
- Advice from an endocrinologist should be sought as soon as possible.

Disability

- In reality this will be assessed prior to treating the hypercalcaemia. It is vital to determine if there is any cognitive impairment, acute psychosis or altered level of consciousness prior to treatment as this aids assessment of severity.

Exposure

If not already done:

- Take a full history and detailed physical assessment.
- Look carefully for any obvious cause of hypercalcaemia if not yet known.

HYPONATRAEMIA

DEFINITION

Hyponatraemia is a serum sodium of <125 mmol/l. One of the most common causes of hyponatraemia is medication. Diuretics, particularly thiazide diuretics, can cause hyponatraemia. However it is important to exclude other causes.

SYMPTOMS AND SIGNS

Patients with hyponatraemia may present with:

- confusion
- oedema
- weight loss
- nausea
- muscle weakness
- shortness of breath due to cardiac failure
- seizures

ASSESSMENT

As always, use an ABCDE approach.

Airway

- Assess and maintain airway.
- Utilise head tilt, chin lift if necessary.
- Use airway adjuncts if required.
- Consider urgent referral to anaesthetist for intubation if unable to protect airway.

Breathing

- Assess oxygen saturations using pulse oximeter – aim to maintain saturations at >92%.
- Give high-flow oxygen via non re-breath mask.
- Assess respiratory rate.
- Examine respiratory system.
- Request chest x-ray – look for signs of heart failure.

Circulation

- Assess heart rate and rhythm.
- Record blood pressure.
- Gain IV access.
- Obtain venous blood for serum sodium, U&E, FBC and glucose.
- Obtain an ECG.
- Obtain urine sample for urinary sodium.
- Assess JVP.
- Assess for signs of dehydration.
- Give slow IV fluids – 0.9% normal saline, aim to increase serum sodium to 125 mmol/l.
- IV furosemide may be given if signs of heart failure are present.
- Seek expert assistance.

Disability

- Assess using AVPU.
- Record blood glucose.
- Treat seizures symptomatically (see Chapter 9).
- Consider restricting fluids to 1 litre a day.

Exposure

If not already done:

- Take a full history and detailed physical assessment.
- Look carefully for any obvious cause of hyponatraemia if not yet known.
- Withhold thiazide diuretics.

SYNDROME OF INAPPROPRIATE ADH SECRETION (SIADH)

SIADH is a recognised cause of hyponatraemia but is frequently misdiagnosed. SIADH is characterised by concentrated urine (sodium >20 mmol/l and osmolality >100 mosm/l) in the presence of hyponatraemia, or low plasma osmolality and the absence of hypovolaemia, oedema or diuretics.

The most common causes of SIADH are malignancies, stroke, subarachnoid haemorrhage, sub-dural haemorrhage, tuberculosis and pneumonia.

The treatment is as for hyponatraemia. Ensure you identify and treat the cause.

HYPERNATRAEMIA

DEFINITION

Hypernatraemia is defined as a serum sodium of >150 mmol/l.

Hypernatraemia is usually caused by water loss in excess of sodium loss. On occasions it can be found to be due to an excessive intake of sodium.

Hypernatraemia occurs in the elderly or those with a decreased level of consciousness when they are unable to take water orally. The body's normal response to thirst may be reduced or absent due to confusion or unconsciousness. Patients who have diarrhoea and do not replace fluid loss can become hypernatraemic as can those who sweat profusely, for example during excessive heat combined with an illness or due to over exertion.

Hypernatraemia can be caused by:

- fluid loss without water replacement
- excessive normal saline given intravenously
- diabetes insipidous – suspect this if the patient is passing large volumes of urine
- osmotic diuresis
- primary aldosteronism – suspect this if the patient is hypertensive, has a low potassium and alkolosis

SYMPTOMS AND SIGNS

Patients with hypernatraemia may present with:

- thirst
- confusion

- lethargy
- seizures
- they may be dehydrated with:
  - dry skin
  - decreased skin turgor
  - postural hypotension
  - oliguria
- blood tests may reveal a raised albumin and urea

ASSESSMENT

As always, utilise an ABCDE approach to assessment.

Airway

- Assess and maintain airway.
- Utilise head tilt, chin lift if necessary.
- Use airway adjuncts if required.
- Consider urgent referral to anaesthetist for intubation if unable to protect airway.

Breathing

- Assess oxygen saturations using pulse oximeter – aim to maintain saturations at >92%.
- Give high-flow oxygen via non re breath mask.
- Assess respiratory rate.
- Examine respiratory system.
- Request chest x-ray.

Circulation

- Assess heart rate and rhythm.
- Record blood pressure.
- Gain IV access.
- Obtain venous blood for serum sodium, U&E, FBC and glucose.
- Obtain an ECG.
- Obtain urine sample for urinary sodium.
- Assess JVP – is the patient normovolaemic or hypovolaemic?
- If the patient is hypovolaemic and asymptomatic:
  - encourage oral fluids
  - monitor serum sodium daily.
- If the patient is hypovolaemic and symptomatic:
  - administer IV 0.9% sodium chloride 1 l over 2–4 hours as this causes less marked fluid shift and is hypotonic in hypernatraemic patients

➢ further IV fluid should be 5% dextrose
➢ do not administer hypotonic fluid IV.
- If the patient's normovolaemic and symptomatic:
    ➢ estimate the patient's water deficit by calculating the patient's ideal body weight (Figure 8.1) and then follow the water deficit calculation in Figure 8.2
    ➢ aim to replace 50% of the patient's water deficit with IV 5% dextrose in the first 24 hours
    ➢ monitor serum sodium every 12 hours.
- Do not allow serum sodium to fall by >10 mmol/l in a 24 hour period.
- Seek expert assistance.

Males:
IBW = 50 + (2.3 × height in inches − 60)
Females:
IBW = 45 + (2.3 × height in inches − 60)
1 cm = 0.394 inches

Figure 8.1. Calculation of ideal body weight.

$$\frac{0.6 \times \text{ideal body weight} \times (\text{serum sodium} - 140)}{140}$$

Figure 8.2. Calculation of water deficit.

Disability

- Assess using AVPU.
- Record blood glucose.
- Treat seizures symptomatically (see Chapter 9).

Exposure

If not already done:

- Take a full history and detailed physical assessment.
- Look carefully for any obvious cause of hypernatraemia if not yet known.
- Treat any underlying cause.

HYPOKALAEMIA

DEFINITION

Hypokalaemia is defined as a serum potassium of <3.5 mmol/l.
   The most common causes of hypokalaemia are:

- diuretic treatment
- hyperaldosteronism
- diarrhoea and vomiting
- renal tubular failure
- Cushing's syndrome
- Conn's syndrome
- pyloric stenosis
- occasionally found to be due to venous blood being taken from a limb with an IV line in situ

SYMPTOMS AND SIGNS

Patients with hypokalaemia are often asymptomatic. However they may present with:

- muscle weakness
- cramps
- hypotonia
- cardiac arrhythmias

ASSESSMENT

As always, utilise an ABCDE approach to assessment.

Airway

- Assess and maintain airway.
- Utilise head tilt, chin lift if necessary.
- Use airway adjuncts if required.
- Consider urgent referral to anaesthetist for intubation if unable to protect airway.

Breathing

- Assess oxygen saturations using pulse oximeter – aim to maintain saturations at >92%.
- Give high-flow oxygen via non re-breath mask.
- Assess respiratory rate.
- Examine respiratory system.
- Request chest x-ray.

Circulation

- Assess heart rate and rhythm.
- Record blood pressure.
- Gain IV access.

- Obtain venous blood for serum potassium in a lithium heparin tube, U&E, FBC, glucose and magnesium level.
- Obtain an arterial blood gas:
  - ➢ look for a metabolic alkalosis
  - ➢ suspect renal tubular acidosis if HC03 <22 mol/l.
- If renal tubular acidosis suspected, refer to renal team urgently.
- Obtain an ECG – look for ST depression, flat T waves, U waves and arrhythmias.
- If there are any adverse cardiac signs, place patient on a cardiac monitor.
- If the patient has adverse cardiac signs, pre-existing cardiac disease or serum potassium is <3.0 mmol/l administer IV 0.9% sodium chloride 500 mls with 20 mmols potassium chloride (KCl) over two hours.
- Repeat serum potassium after IV administered and repeat IV fluids if level remains <3.0 mmol/l or patient continues to have adverse clinical signs.
- If arrhythmias persist despite IV fluid with potassium chloride, refer urgently to cardiology.
- If serum potassium is <3.0 mmol/l and patient is asymptomatic, replace potassium with Sando-K two tablets three times daily for two days.
- If serum potassium is 3.0–3.5 mmol/l and the patient is on digoxin, administer Sando-K three times daily for two days.

Disability

- Assess using AVPU.
- Record blood glucose.

Exposure

If not already done:

- Take a full history and detailed physical assessment.
- Look carefully for any obvious cause of hypokalaemia if not yet known.
- Treat any underlying cause.

HYPERKALAEMIA

DEFINITION

Hyperkalaemia is defined as a serum potassium >6 mmol/l.
   The most common causes of hyperkalaemia are:

- drug therapy such as potassium sparing diuretics and ACE inhibitors
- renal failure
- Addison's disease
- metabolic acidosis
- large volume blood transfusion

- excessive potassium therapy
- rhabdomyolysis

SYMPTOMS AND SIGNS

Frequently the first time a patient knows they have hyperkalaemia is when they suffer a cardiac arrest and this should always be considered as a cause of cardiac arrest (see Chapter 2). Sometimes hyperkalaemia is detected before cardiac arrest occurs. In these cases the patient may present with:

- muscle weakness
- paralysis
- Kussmaul's breathing due to metabolic acidosis
- cardiac arrhythmias

ASSESSMENT

As always, utilise an ABCDE approach to assessment.

Airway

- Assess and maintain airway.
- Utilise head tilt, chin lift if necessary.
- Use airway adjuncts if required.
- Consider urgent referral to anaesthetist for intubation if unable to protect airway.

Breathing

- Assess oxygen saturations using pulse oximeter – aim to maintain saturations at >92%.
- Give high-flow oxygen via non re-breath mask.
- Assess respiratory rate.
- Examine respiratory system.
- Request chest x-ray.

Circulation

- Assess heart rate and rhythm.
- Record blood pressure.
- Gain IV access.
- Obtain venous blood for serum potassium in a lithium heparin tube, U&E, FBC and glucose.
- Obtain an arterial blood gas – look for a metabolic acidosis.

- Obtain an ECG – look for tall tented T waves, flat P waves, increased PR interval and widening of the QRS complex – there is a danger that this can lead to a VF arrest or Torsades de Pointes.
- If there are any adverse cardiac signs, place patient on a cardiac monitor.
- If the patient has adverse cardiac signs:
  - ➤ administer 10 mls of 10% calcium gluconate IV over 5 minutes;
  - ➤ repeat serum potassium level.
- Commence IV infusion of 10 units of actrapid insulin in 50 mls of 50% glucose over 10 minutes – this must be given through a large vein.
- This infusion can be followed by 1 litre of 5% dextrose IV over 12 hours.
- Repeat serum potassium.
- If serum potassium remains elevated, seek medical assistance immediately.
- There may be an indication to commence calcium resonium or to repeat the treatment already given – this should be done under expert guidance.
- If the patient has severe adverse cardiac signs, nebulised salbutamol 2.5 mg can be given back to back to drive potassium into the cells.
- Monitor urine output.

Disability

- Assess using AVPU.
- Record blood glucose.

Exposure

If not already done:

- Take a full history and detailed physical assessment.
- Look carefully for any obvious cause of hyperkalaemia if not yet known.
- Treat any underlying cause.

ADDISONIAN CRISIS

DEFINITION

An Addisonian crisis is defined as an acute onset of adrenocortical insufficiency or the sudden worsening of Addison's disease. It is mainly associated with an acute deficiency of the glucocoticoid cortisol and to a lesser extent the mineralcorticoid aldosterone.

Crisis occurs when the physiological demand for these hormones exceeds the ability of the adrenal gland to produce them. It is a potentially fatal condition if left untreated.

The commonest causes of Addisonian crisis are:

- abrupt withdrawal of steroids
- infection

- injury and trauma such as burns
- surgery
- pregnancy
- administration of general anaesthesia
- physiological stress such as myocardial infarction

SYMPTOMS AND SIGNS

The patient with Addisonian crisis may present with the following:

- confusion
- profound weakness
- abdominal pain
- tachycardia
- hypotension – particularly postural hypotension
- peripheral vasoconstriction
- nausea
- vomiting
- hypoglycaemia
- pyrexia
- hyperpigmentation of the buccal mucosa, pressure points and skin creases may also be noticed
- vitiligo
- absence of body hair

ASSESSMENT

As always use an ABCDE approach. Remember this is a clinical emergency.

Airway

- Assess and maintain airway.
- Utilise head tilt, chin lift if necessary.
- Use airway adjuncts if required.
- Consider urgent referral to anaesthetist for intubation if unable to protect airway.

Breathing

- Assess oxygen saturations using pulse oximeter – aim to maintain saturations at >92%.
- Give high flow oxygen via non re-breath mask.
- Assess respiratory rate.
- Examine respiratory system.
- Request chest x-ray.

Circulation

- Summon medical help.
- Assess heart rate and rhythm.
- Record blood pressure.
- Gain IV access.
- Administer IV fluids:
  - ➤ give 500 mls of Gelofusine if patient is hypotensive;
  - ➤ if hypoglycaemia is present, give 100 mls of 20% dextrose over 30 minutes;
  - ➤ follow this infusion with 1 litre of 10% dextrose over 12 hours.
- Obtain venous blood for U&E, FBC and glucose, cortisol and ACTH.
- Monitor blood glucose using capillary sample.
- Obtain an ECG.
- Insert urinary catheter and monitor output hourly if patient is unconscious or does not pass urine within three hours of starting IV fluids.
- Record patient's temperature.
- Obtain a MSU for culture.
- If the patient is pyrexial obtain blood cultures.
- If possible obtain a sputum sample for culture.
- Administer hydrocortisone 100 mg IV stat – do not wait for the blood tests to confirm the diagnosis. If you suspect an Addisonian crisis start treatment immediately.
- Repeated doses of hydrocortisone 100 mg IV every six hours will be required.
- Consider the need for a broad spectrum antibiotic.

Disability

- Assess using AVPU.
- Monitor blood glucose using capillary sample if not already done.

Exposure

- Once the patient is stable a full detailed history can be obtained.
- If the cause of the crisis has not already been found, look for it now.
- Refer to an endocrinologist.

THYROID CRISIS (THYROID STORM)

DEFINITION

Thyroid crisis is a systemic syndrome that occurs as a result of excess production and release of the thyroid hormones thyroxine and triiodothyronine. A hypermetabolic state occurs as a result of tissue response to an excess of circulating thyroid hormones, causing an increase in cellular function.

Thyrotoxicosis is an all-inclusive term used to describe severe hypermetabolic states that are induced by thyroid hormones. Thyroid crisis occurs when the metabolic, cardiovascular and thermoregulatory mechanisms that have previously been compensating for this hypermetablioc state fail. If this thyroid crisis is untreated, death can occur. It is therefore vital that prompt action is taken.

Some precipitating events that can lead to a thyroid crisis are:

- withdrawal of antithyroid drug therapy
- infection
- sepsis
- trauma
- surgery
- hypoglycaemia
- diabetic ketoacidosis
- pulmonary embolism
- cerebrovascular accident
- seizures
- childbirth
- radioactive iodine therapy

SYMPTOMS AND SIGNS

Patients with thyroid crisis present with the following:

- palpitations
- shortness of breath
- diarrhoea
- jaundice
- weight loss
- restlessness
- tremor
- they may complain of a short attention span and emotional lability
- the patient may have a palpable goitre and be exophthalamous
- confusion
- fever
- coma

ASSESSMENT

As always, use an ABCDE approach.

Airway

- Assess and maintain airway.
- Utilise head tilt, chin lift if necessary.

- Use airway adjuncts if required.
- Consider urgent referral to anaesthetist for intubation if unable to protect airway.

Breathing

- Assess oxygen saturations using pulse oximeter – aim to maintain saturations at >92%.
- Give high-flow oxygen via non re-breath mask.
- Assess respiratory rate.
- Examine respiratory system – look for signs of heart failure.
- Request chest x-ray.
- Obtain sputum sample for culture if patient is producing sputum.

Circulation

- Summon medical help if you have not already done so.
- Assess heart rate and rhythm.
- Record blood pressure.
- Gain IV access.
- Obtain venous blood for U&E, FBC, glucose and Thyroid Function Tests (TFTs).
- Monitor blood glucose using capillary sample.
- Obtain an ECG – look for fast AF.
- Maintain strict fluid balance chart.
- Record patient's temperature.
- Obtain a MSU for culture.
- If the patient is pyrexial obtain blood cultures.
- Administer propanolol 40–80 mg orally depending on local policy – get expert help.
- Carbimazole may be given under expert guidance.
- Treat any heart failure (Chapter 6).
- Consider the need for IV fluids if no signs of heart failure and patient has a pyrexia.
- Consider the need for a broad spectrum antibiotic.

Disability

- Assess using AVPU
- Monitor blood glucose using capillary sample if not already done
- If patient is unable to tolerate oral medication consider passing a nasogastric tube (NG tube).

Exposure

- Once the patient is stable a full detailed history can be obtained.
- If the cause of the crisis has not already been found look for it now.
- Refer to an endocrinologist.

MYXEDEMA CRISIS

DEFINITION

Myxedema coma is a severe life-threatening sequela of profound hypothyroidism. The patient will usually have a history of hypothyroidism or precipitating signs and symptoms suggestive of hypothyroidism. The disease usually evolves from a state of uncomplicated hypothyroidism into central nervous system depression leading to coma. Left untreated there is a high mortality rate.

Factors that may lead to an underlying hypothyroidism suddenly decompensating include:

- hypothermia
- infection
- cerebrovascular accident
- hypoglycaemia
- hyponatraemia
- hypoxaemia
- hypercapnia
- trauma
- drugs such as anaesthetics, sedatives, narcotics and amiodarone
- gastrointestinal bleeding

SYMPTOMS AND SIGNS

Patients with myxedema crisis may present with the following:

- lethargy
- confusion
- hypoventilation
- shortness of breath
- abdominal pain
- constipation
- nausea
- non-pitting oedema
- coma
- signs of dry, coarse scaly skin and sparse or coarse hair

ASSESSMENT

As always, use an ABCDE approach.

Airway

- Assess and maintain airway.
- Utilise head tilt, chin lift if necessary.

- Use airway adjuncts if required.
- Consider urgent referral to anaesthetist for intubation if unable to protect airway – ventilatory support is often required.

Breathing

- Assess oxygen saturations using pulse oximeter – aim to maintain saturations at >92%.
- Give high flow oxygen via non re-breath mask.
- Assess respiratory rate.
- Examine respiratory system – look for signs of heart failure.
- Request chest x-ray.
- Obtain sputum sample for culture if patient is producing sputum.

Circulation

- Summon medical help if you have not already done so.
- Assess heart rate and rhythm.
- Record blood pressure.
- Gain IV access.
- Obtain venous blood for U&E, FBC, glucose and Thyroid Function Tests (TFTs).
- Monitor blood glucose using capillary sample.
- Obtain an ECG.
- Maintain strict fluid balance chart.
- Record patient's temperature.
- If the patient is hypothermic give warmed IV fluids slowly – 5% dextrose over 8 hours.
- If hypothermic gradually re-warm (see Chapters 2 and 11).
- Pass a urinary catheter.
- Obtain a MSU for culture.
- Treat any heart failure (see Chapter 6).
- Consider the need for a broad spectrum antibiotic.
- Give hydrocortisone 100 mg IV eight-hourly.
- IV T3 should be administered, dose depends on patient's age and co-morbidities; gain expert advice before commencing this.

Disability

- Assess using AVPU.
- Monitor blood glucose using capillary sample if not already done.
- If patient is unable to tolerate oral medication consider passing a nasogastric tube (NG tube).
- Once results of U&E are known – if patient is hyponatraemic it is important to correct this in order to improve mental state.

Exposure

- Once the patient is stable a full, detailed history can be obtained.
- If the cause of the crisis has not already been found, look for it now.
- Refer to an endocrinologist urgently for further investigation and advice on thyroid replacement therapy.

REFERENCES

Bradley K, Hammersley M, Levy J, Matthews D and Wallace T (2002) *Guidelines for the Management of Diabetic Hyperosmolar Non-Ketotic State*. Oxford: Oxford Centre for Diabetes, Endocrinology and Metabolism.

Dahlen R (2002) Managing patients with acute thyrotoxicosis. *Critical Care Nurse* 22: 62–9.

Gross P, Wehrle R and Bussemaker E (1996) Hyponatraemia: pathophysiology, differential diagnosis and new aspects of treatment. *Clinical Nephrology* 46(4): 273–6.

Hahner S and Allolio B (2005) Management of adrenal insufficiency in different clinical settings. *Expert Opinion in Pharmacotherapy* Nov 6(14): 2407–17.

Kumar P and Clark M (2003) *Clinical Medicine*, 3rd edn. London: Saunders.

Longmore M, Wilkinson I and Török E (2001) *Oxford Handbook of Clinical Medicine*, 5th edn. Oxford: Oxford University Press.

Malmberg K, Ryden L, Efendic S, Herlitz J, Nicol P, Waldenstrom A et al. (1995) Randomised trial of insulin-glucose infusion followed by subcutaneous insulin treatment in diabetic patients with acute myocardial infarction (DIGAMI study) effects on mortality at 1 year. *Journal of American College of Cardiology* 26: 57–65.

Mesotten D and van den Berhe G (2003) Clinical potential of insulin therapy in critically ill patients. *Drugs* 63(7). 625–36.

National Institute for Clinical Excellence (2004) Type 1 diabetes: diagnosis and management of type 1 diabetes in adults. *Clinical Guideline* 15. London: NICE.

Van den Berghe G, Wouters P, Weekers F, Vrewaest C, Bruyninckx F, Scetz M et al. (2001) Intensive insulin therapy in the critically ill patient. *New England Journal of Medicine* Nov 8 345(19): 1359–67.

9   Neurological Conditions

Neurological emergencies frequently present themselves in the Medical Assessment Unit. Prompt assessment, immediate treatment and referral to a specialist are vital. This chapter details the management of the most commonly presenting neurological emergencies.

STATUS EPILEPTICUS

Status epilepticus is life-threatening, requiring prompt assessment and treatment. It is categorised into four stages:

- 1st stage (0–10 minutes) – early status
- 2nd stage (0–30 minutes) – early status
- 3rd stage (0–60 minutes) – established status
- 4th stage (30–90 minutes) – refractory status

The early intervention of a neurologist is paramount. NICE issued guidance on the management of status epilepticus in 2004. This guidance can be found at www.nice.org.uk

DEFINITION

A state of seizure activity lasting for thirty minutes, or repeated seizures with no return of consciousness. Sixty per cent of all episodes occur in patients without any history of epilepsy (Kumar and Clark 2003). Mortality and the risk of brain damage increase with the length of the attack.

SYMPTOMS AND SIGNS

- seizure activity lasting for 30 minutes with no return of consciousness
- repeated seizures with no return of consciousness between seizures

It will not be possible to obtain information from the patient. Ask relatives/friends:

- Has there been a previous diagnosis of epilepsy?
- Has the patient been in status before?
- Has the patient recently changed their medication?

- Has the patient omitted to take their anti-convulsants recently?
- Has the patient had a recent cold, respiratory tract infection or urinary tract infection?
- Has the patient been suffering from diarrhoea and vomiting prior to admission?
- Is there a history of alcohol abuse?

ASSESSMENT

This is a life-threatening event and prompt management is vital. As always, utilise an ABCDE approach.

Airway

- Summon medical assistance immediately.
- Assess and maintain airway.
- Utilise head tilt, chin lift if necessary.
- Use airway adjuncts if required.
- Consider urgent referral to an anaesthetist if unable to protect the airway as rapid sequence induction is likely to be required.
- Assist breathing with bag valve mask ventilation if the patient is not making adequate respiratory effort (respiration rate <8 per minute).

Breathing

- Give high-flow oxygen via non re-breath mask.
- Assess oxygen saturations using pulse oximeter – aim to maintain saturations at >92%.
- Assess respiratory rate.
- A full respiratory examination is not needed at this stage. This can be performed once the initial emergency is dealt with.
- Request a chest x-ray to evaluate the possibility of aspiration.

Circulation

- Obtain IV access – two large-bore cannulae are advised.
- Obtain venous blood for FBC, U&E, LFTs, INR, calcium and magnesium.
- Save a sample of venous blood for possible toxicology screening at a later date.
- If patient is taking anti-convulsants, send venous blood sample to assess whether levels are therapeutic.
- Commence cardiac monitoring.
- Monitor BP and pulse.
- Obtain arterial blood gases to assess acidosis and oxygenation. If pH <7.0 refer immediately to ITU.
- Insert urinary catheter.
- Obtain a MSU.

- Obtain urine sample for possible toxicology screen at a later date.
- Record blood sugar.
- If any suggestion of alcohol abuse administer 50 mls of 50% glucose IV and commence high potency IV Pabrinex.

Drug therapy is dependent on the stage of status (NICE 2004).

1st and 2nd stage – early status

- Administer IV Lorazepam 0.1 mg/kg.
- Usually give a 4 mg bolus.
- This can be repeated once after 10–20 minutes.
- If the patient is already prescribed anti-convulsants these should be continued as soon as they are able to take them.

3rd stage – established status

- Administer phenytoin infusion at a dose of 15–18 mg/kg at a rate of 50 mg/minute.
- An alternative to this is fosphenytoin infusion at a dose of 15–20 mg phenytoin equivalents (PE)/kg at a rate of 50–100 PE/minute.
- If these are not suitable/available phenobarbitone bolus of 10–15 mg/kg at a rate of 100 mg/minute can be administered.

4th stage – refractory status

- At this stage get an anaesthetist as general anaesthesia is required.
- NICE (2004) recommend the use of one of the following drugs at this stage:
  - ➢ Propofol 1–2 mg/kg bolus followed by 2–10 mg/kg/hour titrated to effect
  - ➢ Midazolam 0.1–0.2 mg/kg bolus followed by 0.05–0.5 mg/kg/hour titrated to effect
  - ➢ Thiopentone 3–5 mg/kg bolus followed by 3–5 mg/kg/hour titrated to effect, with rate reduction after 2–3 days.

Disability

- Assess AVPU – by definition status patients will be unconscious initially.
- Continue to assess using Glasgow Coma Scale or AVPU as condition changes/improves.
- Consider the need for urgent CT scan of the brain.
- Consider the need for urgent lumbar puncture.
- Refer for EEG as soon as possible.

Exposure

- As soon as the patient is stable a full examination can be undertaken.
- Look for signs of injuries that may have been sustained during seizures and document these.
- Establish cause of status epilepticus if not already known.

STROKE

DEFINITION

Stroke is the third most common cause of death in the UK (2002 data, published in Office of National Statistics 2004). It is defined as a focal neurological deficit lasting longer than 24 hours. Both cerebral infarction and intraparenchymal haemorrhage are covered by this definition.

SYMPTOMS AND SIGNS

The area of brain affected by a stroke will determine the symptoms and signs. There are four syndromes encompassed by the term stroke. They are:

Total Anterior Circulation Syndrome (TACS)

- new higher cerebral dysfunction which manifests itself as:
  - ➤ dysphasia
  - ➤ dyscalcullia
  - ➤ visiospatial disorder
  - ➤ homonymous visual field defect
- ipsilateral motor and/or sensory deficit of at least two areas of the face, arm and leg

Partial Anterior Circulation Syndrome (PACS)

- motor and/or sensory deficit restricted to face or arm or leg
- patients presenting with only two of the three components of TACS

Lacunar Syndrome (LACS)

- pure motor, sensory or sensori–motor deficit
- ataxic hemiparesis

Posterior Circulation Syndrome (POCS)

- ipsilateral cranial nerve palsy
- contralateral motor and/or sensory deficit
- bilateral motor and/or sensory deficit
- disorder of conjugate eye movement
- cerebellar dysfunction without ipsilateral hemiparesis
- isolated homonymous visual field defect

ASSESSMENT

As always, use an ABCDE approach.

Airway

- Assess and maintain airway.
- Utilise head tilt, chin lift if necessary.
- Use airway adjuncts if required.
- Assist breathing with bag valve mask ventilation if patient not making adequate respiratory effort (respiration rate <8 per minute).

Breathing

- Give high flow oxygen via non re-breath mask.
- Assess oxygen saturations using pulse oximeter – aim to maintain saturations at >92%.
- Assess respiratory rate.
- Undertake a respiratory examination.
- Request a chest x-ray.

Circulation

- Obtain IV access.
- Obtain venous blood for FBC, U&E, LFTs, INR, CRP, ESR and random cholesterol.
- Record ECG.
- Monitor BP and pulse – do not attempt to lower BP acutely unless >220/120 mmHg.
- Give sodium chloride 0.9% 1 litre over six hours if consciousness impaired or patient dehydrated.
- Monitor BM – if blood sugar >11 mmol/l consider using insulin to maintain glycaemic control.
- Monitor temperature – treat pyrexia with paracetamol 1 g and consider broad spectrum antibiotics.
- Do not catheterise unless the patient is in urinary retention.

Disability

- Assess using AVPU.
- If consciousness decreased place nil by mouth.
- Thrombolysis may be indicated. This is not offered by all hospitals – know your local policies.
- Refer for urgent CT scan.

- If time of onset of symptoms is known and it is within two hours, the patient may be a candidate for thrombolysis.
- Thrombolysis is usually in the form of tPA. The dose is 0.9 mg/kg over 60 minutes; 10% of dose is given within the first minute.

Exposure

- Undertake a full neurological examination.
- Assess swallowing if not already done.
- Refer to a stroke specialist as the patient is going to require a multi-disciplinary team assessment and management in order to aid recovery.

TRANSIENT ISCHAEMIC ATTACKS (TIA)

DEFINITION

TIAs are usually the result of the passage of microemboli which lyse, arising from atheromatous plaques or cardiac mural thrombi (Kumar and Clark 2003). A TIA is characterised by an acute loss of focal cerebral or ocular function with symptoms lasting less than 24 hours.

SYMPTOMS AND SIGNS

Features of TIA depend on the arterial territory affected. The two territories are the carotid and the vertebrobasilar systems. Symptoms and signs for each system are:

Carotid system

- amaurosis fugax – the sudden loss of vision in one eye as a result of the passage of emboli through the retinal arteries
- aphasia
- hemiparesis
- hemisensory loss
- hemianopic visual loss

Vertebrobasilar system

- diplopia
- vertigo
- vomiting
- choking
- dysarthria
- ataxia

- hemisensory loss
- hemianopic visual loss
- transient global amnesia
- loss of consciousness

ASSESSMENT

As always, use an ABCDE approach.

Airway

- Assess and maintain airway.
- Utilise head tilt, chin lift if necessary.
- Use airway adjuncts if required.

Breathing

- Assess oxygen saturations using pulse oximeter – aim to maintain saturations at >92%.
- Give high-flow oxygen via non re-breath mask if oxygen saturations <92%.
- Assess respiratory rate.
- Undertake a respiratory examination.
- Request a chest x-ray.

Circulation

- Obtain IV access.
- Obtain venous blood for FBC, U&E, LFTs, INR, ESR and random cholesterol.
- Record ECG – if in AF consider anticoagulation.
- Listen for a carotid bruit.
- Listen to heart sounds for signs of a murmur.
- Monitor BP and pulse – do not attempt to lower BP acutely unless >220/120 mmHg.
- Monitor BM

Disability

- Assess using AVPU.
- Refer for a CT scan to exclude haemorrhage – this may be as an in-patient or an out-patient depending on local policies.
- Once a haemorrhage is excluded, give aspirin 75 mg orally daily.
- Refer for a carotid Doppler.
- Consider referral for echocardiography if in AF or a murmur is found on examination.

Exposure

- Undertake a full neurological examination.
- Know your local policies – many hospitals have TIA clinics and patients should be referred to them for follow-up.
- Patients who have suffered a TIA should refrain from driving for one month.
- After one month they can resume driving without notifying DVLA, providing they have made a satisfactory clinical recovery.

ISOLATED SEIZURE AND UNEXPLAINED LOSS OF CONSCIOUSNESS

DEFINITION

An episode of loss of consciousness with or without convulsive movement. The best account is from an eye witness.

SYMPTOMS AND SIGNS

This is a common clinical presentation to the MAU. Many of these patients will have normal investigations and be discharged home directly from MAU. However, it is important to ensure a thorough history and examination is undertaken as occasionally you will detect something abnormal which warrants further investigation and treatment.

Common causes of altered levels of consciousness are:

- syncope – this can include:
  - ➢ simple faint
  - ➢ cough syncope
  - ➢ micturition syncope
- cardiac arrhythmias
- postural hypotension
- epilepsy
- hypoglycaemia
- transient ischaemic attacks
- panic attacks
- hyperventilation
- narcolepsy
- cataplexy

ASSESSMENT

As always, use an ABCDE approach.

Airway

- Assess and maintain airway.
- Utilise head tilt, chin lift if necessary.
- Use airway adjuncts if required.

Breathing

- Assess oxygen saturations using pulse oximeter – aim to maintain saturations at >92%.
- Give high flow oxygen via non re-breath mask if oxygen saturations <92%.
- Assess respiratory rate.
- Undertake a respiratory examination.
- Request a chest x-ray.

Circulation

- Obtain IV access.
- Obtain venous blood for FBC, U&E and glucose.
- Record ECG.
- Listen for carotid bruit.
- Listen to heart sounds for signs of a murmur.
- Monitor BP and pulse.
- Monitor BM.

Disability

- Assess using AVPU.
- Undertake a neurological examination.
- If there is a focal neurological deficit then refer for an urgent CT head.

Exposure

- If not already obtained, gain an eye witness account of events.
- Establish history of previous episodes.
- Establish if there is a history of early morning jerks or absence episodes.
- Establish if there is a previous history of treated epilepsy.
- If all investigations are normal then patient can be discharged home.
- If abnormal investigations – refer to appropriate speciality for follow up.
- Following an isolated seizure the patient should be advised not to drive for one year.
- They must be told that they need to inform the DVLA.
- After one year if there have been no further seizures they may regain their licence subject to a medical review.
- Ensure this is documented in the medical notes.

HEADACHE

DEFINITION

The dictionary definition is 'a pain in the head'. Headache is a common presenting problem, both in primary and secondary care. It is important that practitioners can differentiate between the headache that is self-limiting and of no major concern and that which is disabling and a symptom of a serious underlying condition. Headaches can be classified as follows:

- acute single episode
- acute recurrent headache
- subacute in onset
- chronic headache

For each classification certain diagnoses are more prevalent:

Acute single episode

- meningitis
- subarachnoid haemorrhage
- encephalitis
- following head injury
- secondary to medication (e.g. GTN headache)

Acute recurrent attacks

- migraine
- cluster headache
- glaucoma

Subacute in onset

- giant cell arteritis

Chronic headache

- tension headache
- headache related to continuing use of analgesia
- chronically raised intra cranial pressure (ICP)

When assessing a patient with a headache the most important information is in the history. It is important that you let the patient tell you about their headache and the chronological order in which symptoms manifested themselves.

In place of a list of symptoms and signs, what follows is the typical presentation for the common causes of headache:

- *Meningitis* – acute, severe and felt all over the head (see Chapter 4, Infection).

- *Subarachnoid haemorrhage* – acute, severe and felt all over the head (covered later in this chapter).
- *Encephalitis* – acute, severe and felt all over the head. It may be associated with fever and seizures.
- *Following head injury* – pain may be at the site of injury or more generalised. Always be sure to rule out a subdural haematoma.
- *Secondary to medication (e.g. GTN headache)* – felt very shortly after taking medication. Headache is generalised and usually resolves with analgesia.
- *Migraine* – headache lasting 4–72 hours. The patient may have an aura. It is usually associated with nausea and vomiting and/or photophobia. Patients usually have known triggers for migraine.
- *Cluster headache* – intermittent headache. This is usually nightly pain in one eye. Symptoms last for up to approximately eight weeks and then subside for several months.
- *Glaucoma* – a constant aching pain around one eye. The eyes appear red and the patient has decreased visual acuity.
- *Giant cell arteritis* – headache lasting for a few weeks. This is predominantly a diagnosis in >50 years of age. Tenderness of the scalp is a major complaint and there may be tenderness over the temporal arteries. Visual acuity may be decreased. ESR will be raised. If not treated promptly blindness may occur.
- *Tension headache* – described as a tight band around the head. It may be associated with low mood. On questioning the patient often reveals stress at home or at work.
- *Headache related to continuing use of analgesia* – seen in patients who continually use analgesia, tranquillisers or hypnotics. The intervention of a neurologist is required to manage the chronic problem and the withdrawal of medication.
- *Chronically raised intra cranial pressure (ICP)* – headache upon waking in the morning which improves on sitting up. It is usually associated with nausea and vomiting. Papilloedema, ataxia and altered neurological status require the urgent advice of a neurologist.

ASSESSMENT

As always, use an ABCDE approach.

Airway

- Assess and maintain airway.
- Utilise head tilt, chin lift if necessary.
- Use airway adjuncts if required.

Breathing

- Assess oxygen saturations using pulse oximeter – aim to maintain saturations at >92%.
- Give high-flow oxygen via non re-breath mask if oxygen saturations <92%.
- Assess respiratory rate.
- Undertake a respiratory examination.
- Request a chest x-ray if there are clinical signs of a respiratory problem.

Circulation

- Record BP and pulse.
- Obtain IV access.
- Obtain venous blood for FBC, U&E, glucose and ESR.
- Record ECG.

Disability

- Assess using AVPU.
- Obtain a detailed history of the chronology of events.
- Obtain information pertaining to:
  - time of onset
  - duration of symptoms
  - character of the headache, e.g. dull, stabbing, thunderclap
  - exacerbating and relieving factors
  - associated features, e.g. nausea, vomiting, photophobia, phonophobia, neck stiffness
  - triggers, e.g. cheese, chocolate, alcohol, caffeine, exercise, travel
  - any medication/therapy already tried.
- Undertake a neurological examination.
- If there is a focal neurological deficit then refer for an urgent CT head.
- Consider the need for a lumbar puncture.
- If you have not already done so, seek medical assistance.

Exposure

- If you have not already done so, undertake a detailed physical examination.

SUBARACHNOID HAEMORRHAGE (SAH)

DEFINITION

A subarachnoid haemorrhage is spontaneous arterial bleeding into the subarachnoid space. It is often a catastrophic event and is most commonly seen in the 35–65 age group. SAH accounts for approximately 5% of all strokes and has an annual incidence of 6 per 100,000 (Kumar and Clark 2003).

SAH occurs when:

- a saccular or berry aneurysm ruptures – this accounts for approximately 70% of cases
- a congenital arteriovenous malformation ruptures

In approximately 20% of cases no lesion can be found.
These aneurysms and malformations are usually not detected prior to the rupture which leads to a SAH.

SYMPTOMS AND SIGNS

Patients with a SAH usually present with:

- sudden severe headache frequently occipital – often described as a 'thunderclap' or 'like I've been kicked in the head'
- vomiting
- collapse with loss of consciousness (LOC)
- drowsiness
- coma
- neck stiffness
- hemiplegia
- papilloedema
- retinal and subhyloid haemorrhage

ASSESSMENT

As always, use an ABCDE approach.

Airway

- Assess and maintain airway.
- Utilise head tilt, chin lift if necessary.
- Use airway adjuncts if required.
- Assist breathing with bag valve mask ventilation if patient not making adequate respiratory effort (respiration rate <8 per minute).

Breathing

- Give high-flow oxygen via non re-breath mask.
- Assess oxygen saturations using pulse oximeter – aim to maintain saturations at >92%.
- Assess respiratory rate.

- Undertake a respiratory examination.
- Request a chest x-ray.

Circulation

- Obtain IV access.
- Obtain venous blood for FBC, U&E, LFTs, INR, CRP, ESR and random cholesterol.
- Record ECG.
- Monitor BP and pulse – do not attempt to lower BP acutely unless >220/120 mmHg.
- Give sodium chloride 0.9% 1 litre over eight hours.
- Monitor BM – if blood sugar >11 mmol/l, consider using insulin to maintain glycaemic control.
- Monitor temperature – treat pyrexia with paracetamol 1 g and consider broad spectrum antibiotics.
- Do not catheterise unless the patient is in urinary retention.

Disability

- Assess using AVPU.
- If consciousness decreased place nil by mouth.
- Refer for urgent CT scan – SAH is detected in 95% of cases if CT is done within 24 hours.
- If the CT is normal and clinical suspicion is of a SAH an LP is indicated.
- If you have not already done so, get medical assistance now.
- On performing a LP CSF must be sent to the laboratory to test for the presence of xanthochromia. CSF must be kept in a darkened container and sent to the lab urgently.
- Dexametasone may be useful to reduce cerebral oedema – liaise with neurology and neurosurgery.
- The commencement of a calcium channel blocker such as nimodipine 60 mg four-hourly may help to reduce cerebral artery spasm but should only be commenced on the advice of neurology or neurosurgery.

Exposure

- If you have not already done so, undertake a full clinical examination.
- Urgent referral to the neurosurgeons is required.
- Following a SAH there is a high risk of re-bleeding. Although the patient may survive initially, 10–20% of patient die in the following few weeks.

1

SPINAL CORD COMPRESSION

DEFINITION

Spinal cord compression occurs usually as a result of a neoplasm, lesion or inflammation causing undue pressure on the spinal cord resulting in limb weakness or paralysis.

Acute cord compression is a clinical emergency. Left untreated it may result in irreversible loss of power and sensation below the level of the lesion.

SYMPTOMS AND SIGNS

The patient with spinal cord compression may present with:

- weakness in the arms or legs
- sensory loss
- localised spinal pain and tenderness
- loss of sphincter control
- urinary retention
- erectile dysfunction in men
- constipation – usually in later stages

ASSESSMENT

As always, use an ABCDE approach.

Airway

- Assess and maintain airway.
- Utilise head tilt, chin lift if necessary.
- Use airway adjuncts if required.
- Assist breathing with bag valve mask ventilation if patient not making adequate respiratory effort (respiration rate <8 per minute).

Breathing

- Give high-flow oxygen via non re-breath mask.
- Assess oxygen saturations using pulse oximeter – aim to maintain saturations at >92%.
- Assess respiratory rate.
- Undertake a respiratory examination.
- Request a chest x-ray.

Circulation

- Obtain IV access.

- Obtain venous blood for FBC, U&E, LFTs, INR and ESR.
- Consider the need to send venous blood for PSA and syphilis serology.
- Record temperature.
- If patient pyrexial obtain blood cultures.
- Record BP and pulse.
- Do not catheterise unless the patient is in urinary retention.

Disability

- Assess using AVPU.
- Undertake a full neurological examination.
- Look for a sensory level.
- If you have not already done so, seek medical advice now.
- Refer for an urgent MRI scan – this should include the whole neural axis, cervical, thoracic and lumbar spine.

Exposure

- If you have not already done so, undertake a full clinical examination.
- Urgent referral to the spinal surgeons is required.
- Dexametasone may be useful but should be commenced in conjunction with advice from the spinal surgeons.

REFERENCES

Kumar P and Clark M (2003) *Clinical Medicine*, 3rd edn. London: Saunders.
Loblaw DA, Perry J, Chamber A and Laperriere NJ (2005) Systematic review of the diagnosis and management of malignant extradural spinal cord compression. *Journal of Clinical Oncology* 23: 2028–37.
Longmore M, Wilkinson I and Török E (2001) *Oxford Handbook of Clinical Medicine*, 5th edn. Oxford: Oxford University Press.
National Institute for Clinical Excellence (2004) *The Epilepsies: Diagnosis and Management of the Epilepsies in Adults in Primary and Secondary Care*. Clinical Guideline 20. London: NICE.
Office of National Statistics (2004) *Mortality of Circulatory Diseases 2002*. London: Office of National Statistics.
Royal College of Physicians (2004) *National Clinical Guideline for Stroke*, 2nd edn. Prepared by the Intercollegiate Stroke Working Party. London: Royal College of Physicians.
Siberstein SD and Rosenberg J (2000) Multispeciality consensus on diagnosis and treatment of headache. *Neurology* 54: 1553.

10   Renovascular Conditions

Patients presenting with renovascular conditions will, without doubt, require referral to the renal specialists at an early stage. However, initial management is the responsibility of the MAU team. As a nurse practitioner you must be able to recognise and manage the initial presentation of these conditions before referring for specialist help.

ACUTE RENAL FAILURE (ARF)

DEFINITION

A significant deterioration in renal function occurring over hours or days. It is usually reversible or self-limiting. There is no universally accepted definition of ARF but commonly used definitions include an increase in the serum creatinine of more than 44 mcmol/l or more than 50% over the baseline value (Department of Health 2005).

SYMPTOMS AND SIGNS

ARF can be:

- prerenal – failure of perfusion of the kidneys with blood, most commonly the result of hypotension
- renal – categorised according to the primary site of injury, i.e. tubules, interstitium, renal vessels or glomerulus
- postrenal – both urinary outflow tracts are obstructed; usually easily reversed by relieving the obstruction, e.g. catheterisation

Patients are often asymptomatic in the early stages of ARF. It is only when the plasma urea concentration reaches >40 mmol/l that patients become symptomatic. Patients typically present with:

- alteration of urine volume
  - ➢ oliguria (urine output <30 ml a day)
  - ➢ polyuria (passage of large amounts of dilute urine)
- weakness
- fatigue
- mental confusion
- seizures
- coma – with severe uraemia

- pallor – due to anaemia (more common in chronic renal failure but is seen in ARF)
- pruritus
- bruising due to impaired platelet function
- breathlessness – if anaemic or in pulmonary oedema
- Kussmaul's breathing – sighing respiration due to metabolic acidosis
- nausea and vomiting
- anorexia

ASSESSMENT

As always, use an ABCDE approach.

Airway

- Assess and maintain airway.
- Utilise head tilt, chin lift if necessary.
- Use airway adjuncts if required.
- Consider urgent referral to anaesthetist for intubation if unable to protect airway.

Breathing

- Assess oxygen saturations using pulse oximeter – aim to maintain saturations at >92%.
- Give high-flow oxygen via non re-breath mask if the patient is hypoxic.
- Assess respiratory rate.
- Examine respiratory system.
- Request chest x-ray – looking for signs of pulmonary oedema.

Circulation

- Summon medical assistance as you are likely to need it.
- Assess heart rate and rhythm.
- Record blood pressure.
- Gain IV access.
- Obtain venous blood for U&E, FBC, ESR, plasma protein and urine electrophoresis and consider immunology screen.
- If possible obtain previous U&E results to assess if there is a chronic element to this event.
- Obtain arterial blood gases to assess hypoxia and acidosis.
- Obtain an ECG.
- Assess skin turgor for evidence of dehydration.
- Assess JVP for dehydration/overload.
- If possible record lying and standing BP as indication of dehydration.
- If dehydrated administer IV sodium chloride 0.9%.

- Consider the need for a central venous pressure line – get help if it has not already arrived.
- If the patient remains hypotensive despite rehydration, administer 500 mls of Gelofusine stat.
- If the patient remains hypotensive, inotropes may be indicated – get help now!
- Perform abdominal examination – looking for palpable bladder.
- A strict input/output chart is required.
- Consider inserting a urinary catheter to monitor output hourly.
- Urine dipstick – look for haematuria and/or proteinuria.
- Re-examine the chest looking for signs of fluid overload.
- If clinical evidence of fluid overload give furosemide 250 mg IV over one hour.
- Record patient's temperature.

Disability

- Assess level of consciousness using AVPU.
- Treat any seizures as per Chapter 9.

Exposure

- If you have not already done so – undertake a full history and examination.
- Obtain a detailed drug history.
- Stop any non-steroidal anti-inflammatory drug.
- Stop any nephrotoxic drugs.
- Refer for urgent renal ultrasound to assess size of kidneys and to exclude any obstruction.
- Refer urgently to the renal team for further management.

ACCELERATED (MALIGNANT) HYPERTENSION

DEFINITION

Severe hypertension with evidence of arteriolar damage. It may occur in patients with essential or secondary hypertension. Without effective treatment prognosis is poor, with less than 10% of patients surviving one year. With effective treatment prognosis is good with more than 80% of patients surviving for five years (Webster et al. 1993).

SYMPTOMS AND SIGNS

- headache – the most common presenting complaint
- blurring of vision
- mental impairment – confusion
- dyspnoea – a sign of left ventricular failure

- microscopic haematuria on urinary dipstick
- cotton wool spots on fundoscopy – with or without papilloedema

ASSESSMENT

As always, use an ABCDE approach to assessment.

Airway

- Assess and maintain airway.
- Utilise head tilt, chin lift if necessary.
- Use airway adjuncts if required.

Breathing

- Assess oxygen saturations using pulse oximeter – aim to maintain saturations at >92%.
- Give high-flow oxygen via non re-breath mask if oxygen saturations <92% and no history of COPD.
- Assess respiratory rate.
- Examine respiratory system – look for signs of heart failure.
- Request chest x-ray – looking for signs of pulmonary oedema.

Circulation

- Assess heart rate and rhythm.
- Record blood pressure – take a series of readings.
- If diastolic BP >120 mmHg commence atenolol 50 mg orally once daily or nifedipine SR 10 mg orally twelve-hourly.
- Aim to reduce BP by no more than 25% in the first 48 hours.
- Gain IV access.
- Obtain venous blood for U&E, FBC.
- Obtain an ECG.

Disability

- Assess level of consciousness using AVPU.
- Perform fundoscopy – retinopathy of grade III or IV requires urgent treatment.
- If there is evidence of grade III or IV retinopathy summon help if you have not already done so.

Exposure

- If not already done – undertake a full history and examination.
- Refer urgently to the renal team for further management.

LIFE-THREATENING FEATURES

If any of the following are suspected or present it is vital that you summon medical assistance immediately:

- aortic dissection
- hypertensive encephalopathy
- intracranial haemorrhage
- phaeochromocytoma crisis
- acute pulmonary oedema
- unstable angina
- acute renal insufficiency

These are indications for parenteral therapy. This should only be done under the supervision of expert help. Therefore urgent referral to the renal team is indicated.

The recommended parenteral therapy is IV sodium nitroprusside or labetalol. This is not your remit but that of the experts. Leave them to it.

REFERENCES

Department of Health (2005) *National Service Framework for Renal Services. Part 2: Chronic Kidney Disease, Acute Renal Failure and End of Life Care.* London: DoH.

Longmore M, Wilkinson I and Török E (2001) *Oxford Handbook of Clinical Medicine*, 5th edn. Oxford: Oxford University Press.

National Institute for Clinical Excellence (2004) *Management of Hypertension in Adults.* Clinical Guideline CG018. London: NICE.

Scottish Intercollegiate Guideline Network (2001) *Hypertension in Older People.* Guideline 14. Edinburgh: SIGN.

Webster J, Petrie JC, Jeffers TA and Lovell HG (1993) Accelerated hypertension – patterns of mortality and clinical factors affecting outcome in treated patients. *Quarterly Journal of Medicine* 86: 485–93.

11 Elderly Care

The population is increasing in age. People are living longer, and with that comes the increasing burden on healthcare. Elderly patients presenting to the MAU are likely to have a number of co-morbidities and will therefore have complex needs. These complex needs are best managed by a team of health care professionals who have expertise in this field. However, it is the remit of staff in the MAU to manage the initial acute problem before referring on to the specialists.

HYPOTHERMIA

This has already been covered to some extent in Chapter 2. This section will give more detail in the context of the elderly patient who is hypothermic.

DEFINITION

Hypothermia is defined as the core body temperature falling below 35 °C.

- Mild hypothermia – 35–32 °C
- Moderate hypothermia – 32–30 °C
- Severe hypothermia – less than 30 °C

SYMPTOMS AND SIGNS

When managing a patient who is hypothermic, consider if this is a primary or secondary problem.

- Is hypothermia the main medical problem?
- Has there been another event, for example cardiac arrhythmia, which has caused the patient to collapse and have they then become hypothermic?

In mild hypothermia the patient may not exhibit any signs or complain of feeling cold. As the hypothermia worsens the following may be present:

- shivering
- cold and mottled skin
- swelling of face
- rigid muscles
- depressed respiratory rate

- bradycardia
- hypotension
- confusion
- apathy
- deep reflexes may be absent
- plantars may be extensor
- signs of a precipitating condition may be present

ASSESSMENT

As always, use an ABCDE approach to assessment.

Airway

- Ensure airway is patent.
- Utilise airway adjuncts if necessary.
- Support respiration by bag valve mask ventilation if necessary.
- If the airway is compromised contact anaesthetist and ICU immediately for possible rapid sequence induction (RSI).

Breathing

- Assess respiratory rate.
- Assess oxygen saturations – aim to maintain saturations at >92%.
- Give 100% oxygen via non re-breath mask if saturations <92% and there is no evidence of COPD – oxygen can be warmed.
- If there is evidence of COPD give 24% O_2.
- Obtain arterial blood gases.
- Auscultate chest – listen for signs of infection/failure.
- Request chest x-ray – looking for signs of infection/failure.

Circulation

- Measure core body temperature.
- Assess heart rate and rhythm.
- Monitor blood pressure.
- Record ECG – bradycardia may be present, look for J waves.
- Continuous cardiac monitoring should be initiated.
- Check capillary refill time.
- Gain intravenous access.
- Obtain venous blood for FBC, U&E, TSH, cardiac enzymes and blood glucose.
- Obtain blood cultures.
- Obtain samples of urine and sputum for culture and sensitivity.

- Perform urinalysis.
- Give warmed IV fluids.

Disability

- Assess level of consciousness using AVPU score.

Exposure

- Undertake a full history and examination.
- Look for a cause of hypothermia.
- Gradually re-warm using a space blanket.
- Aim to re-warm at a rate of $1/2°$ an hour.

CONFUSION

DEFINITION

An unexplained change in a patient's mental state and behaviour.

SYMPTOMS AND SIGNS

It is important to remember that confusion is not a diagnosis, it is a symptom. It is important to establish what you are dealing with (Young and George 1995). Is this:

- Delirium (acute confusional state)?
    - ➢ acute confusion in a previously well patient
    - ➢ develops over a few hours or days
- Dementia?
    - ➢ continuing confusion
    - ➢ usually unchanged on presentation
- Delirium superimposed on dementia?
    - ➢ acute confusion in patient with previous cognitive impairment
    - ➢ suddenly becomes much worse
- Acute functional psychosis?
    - ➢ known schizophrenia
    - ➢ parphrenia – commences in patients over the age of 60 years
    - ➢ depression

ASSESSMENT

As always, use an ABCDE approach.

Airway

- Ensure airway is patent.
- Utilise airway adjuncts if necessary.

Breathing

- Assess respiratory rate.
- Assess oxygen saturations.
- Give oxygen if saturations <92% – aim to maintain saturations >92%.
- Auscultate chest – listen for signs of infection/failure.
- Request chest x-ray – look for signs of infection/failure.
- Consider the need for arterial blood gases if hypoxaemia and/or acidosis are suspected as causes of confusion.

Circulation

- Assess heart rate and rhythm.
- Monitor blood pressure.
- Record ECG.
- Gain intravenous access.
- Obtain venous blood for FBC, U&E, calcium, cardiac enzymes, B12, folate and ferritin and blood glucose.
- Obtain blood cultures.
- Obtain samples of urine and sputum for culture and sensitivity.
- Perform urinalysis.
- Correct any electrolyte disturbance.
- Monitor BM and correct hypoglycaemia.

Disability

- Assess level of consciousness using AVPU score.
- Assess confusion using Hodkinson's abbreviated mental test score (1972). See Figure 11.1.
- If the patient is very agitated and disturbed consider sedation.
- Lorazepam 0.5 mg – 1 mg orally or intramuscular to a maximum of 4 mg in 24 hours can be given.
- Alternatively use haloperidol 2.5 mg orally or intramuscular.
- Consider the need for a lumbar puncture.
- Consider referral for EEG.

Exposure

- Undertake a full history and examination.

- If the cause of confusion is not already found, assess for any obvious cause.
- Refer to a specialist care of the elderly team for further assessment.

	Award one point for each correct answer
1.	Age
2.	Time (nearest hour)
3.	An address for recall at the end of the test (this should be repeated by the patient to ensure it has been heard correctly, e.g. 42 West Street)
4.	Year
5.	Name of hospital
6.	Recognition of two persons (doctor, nurse etc.)
7.	Date of birth
8.	Date of World War I
9.	Name of present monarch
10.	Count backwards (20–1)
	A score of seven or less is consistent with impaired brain function

Figure 11.1. Abbreviated Mental Test Score. *Source*: HM Hodkinson (1972) Abbreviated Mental Test Score. *Age and Ageing* 1(4). Reproduced with kind permission of Oxford University Press.

REFERENCES

Department of Health (2001) *National Service Framework for Older People*. London: DoH.

Hodkinson HM (1972) Evaluation of a mental test score for assessment of mental impairment in the elderly. *Age and Ageing* 1(4): 233–8.

Resuscitation Council (2005) *Advanced Life Support Guideline*. London: Resuscitation Council.

Young L and George J (1995) *Guidelines for the Diagnosis and Management of Delirium in the Elderly*. London: British Geriatric Society.

12 Haematological Conditions

The most common haematological condition presenting in the MAU is severe anaemia. Other haematological conditions are rarely seen in the MAU; however, practitioners need to be able to manage the acute presentation of sickle cell crisis and neutropenic sepsis until expert help is available. It is for this reason that these are covered in this chapter. Other haematological conditions require the expert management of haematologists immediately and are therefore not covered in this chapter.

SEVERE ANAEMIA

DEFINITION

Anaemia is defined as a low haemoglobin concentration. An Hb of <8 g/dl is classified as severe anaemia.

There are three different types of anaemia.

Microcytic anaemia – a low MCV

Common causes are:

- iron-deficiency anaemia
- thalassaemia
- congenital sideroblastic anaemia

Normocytic anaemia – normal MCV

Common causes are:

- anaemia of chronic disease
- hypothyroidism
- bone marrow failure
- renal failure
- haemolysis
- pregnancy

Macrocytic anaemia – high MCV

Common causes are:

- B_{12} deficiency
- folate deficiency
- alcohol excess
- liver disease
- cytotoxic drugs
- hypothyroidism
- marrow infiltration
- myelodysplastic syndromes
- reticulocytosis
- antifolate drugs such as phenytoin

SYMPTOMS AND SIGNS

Symptoms depend on the severity and speed of onset of anaemia. Patients may present with the following:

- fatigue
- dyspnoea – particularly on exertion
- anorexia
- headache
- dyspepsia
- altered bowel habit
- increasing frequency and intensity of pre-existing angina
- pallor
- tachycardia
- heart failure
- heart murmur
- cardiac enlargement
- jaundice
- koilonychia (spoon shaped nails)
- spontaneous bruising

ASSESSMENT

As always, use an ABCDE approach.

Airway

- Assess and maintain airway.
- Utilise head tilt, chin lift if necessary.
- Use airway adjuncts if required.

• Consider urgent referral to anaesthetist for intubation if unable to protect airway.

Breathing

• Assess oxygen saturations using pulse oximeter – aim to maintain saturations at >92%.
• Give high-flow oxygen via non re-breath mask if saturations <92% and no history of COPD.
• Assess respiratory rate.
• Examine respiratory system.
• Request chest x-ray.

Circulation

• Assess heart rate and rhythm.
• Record blood pressure.
• Gain IV access.
• Obtain venous blood for group and save, U&E, FBC, LFTs, serum ferritin, B_{12} and folate.
• Obtain venous blood for blood film.
• If possible, obtain previous blood results as this may aid diagnosis.
• Urgent blood transfusion is not indicated unless there is evidence of acute bleeding. In this case see Chapter 7.
• If patient is symptomatic, blood transfusion may aid symptoms.
• If blood is to be administered, give two units of blood, each unit over four hours.
• Give furosemide 20 mg orally with the first unit.

Disability

• Assess conscious level using AVPU.
• Determine type of anaemia if not already done.

Exposure

• If you have not already done so, obtain a detailed history and undertake a full physical examination.
• Ask specifically about:
  ➢ altered bowel habit
  ➢ malaena
  ➢ diet
  ➢ menstrual bleeding
  ➢ other bleeding
  ➢ family history of anaemia.
• If iron deficiency anaemia is present give ferrous sulphate 200 mg three times daily.

- If macrocytic anaemia is present administer hydroxocobalamin 1 mg IM on alternate days for six doses and folic acid 5 mg twice daily.
- If the cause has not been found refer patient for a gastroscopy and possible colonoscopy or barium enema.

SICKLE CELL CRISIS

DEFINITION

Sickle cell disease is a family of inherited haemoglobin disorders. These include sickle cell anaemia (HbSS) and sickle beta thalassaemia (Hb Beta–Thal).

There are over 300 different types of haemoglobin. The most common of these is haemoglobin A. Most people inherit haemoglobin A from both parents (HbAA). Sickle cell trait is present when a person inherits one HbA gene and one HbS gene from their parents. Sickle cell trait cannot therefore develop into sickle cell anaemia. Sickle cell anaemia occurs when a person inherits two HbS genes, one from each parent (HbSS). The incidence of sickle cell disease in Africa is approximately 25%.

Sickle cell crisis occurs when HbS molecules in a deoxygenated state link to form chains which increase the rigidity of the red cells. Premature destruction of the red cells occurs, a process known as haemolysis. This results in occlusion of the microcirculation and infarction of tissue.

Severe sickle cell crisis is life-threatening and therefore requires prompt assessment and management.

SYMPTOMS AND SIGNS

Patients with sickle cell crisis may present with the following:

- severe pain – this may be in the:
  - ➢ chest
  - ➢ abdomen
  - ➢ back
  - ➢ jaw
  - ➢ legs
  - ➢ arms
- lethargy
- pallor
- shortness of breath
- jaundice
- fever
- seizures
- the patient may appear dehydrated

LIFE-THREATENING FEATURES

Sickle cell crisis can and does kill. Three particular concerns that are potentially fatal are:

- acute chest syndrome
- splenic sequestration – death can occur in 30 minutes
- aplastic crisis

Acute chest syndrome

This is characterised by pulmonary infiltrates involving complete lung segments. The chief cause of the infiltrates is fat embolism.

Patients may present with:

- severe chest pain
- fever
- tachypnoea
- wheeze
- cough

Treatment should be on clinical suspicion alone as the syndrome may manifest itself 2–3 days before infiltrates are seen on chest x-ray.

Splenic sequestration

Death from splenic sequestration can occur within 30 minutes. Large amounts of blood become trapped in the spleen. As a result the spleen and liver enlarge rapidly.

The patient may present with:

- severe right upper quadrant pain.

Urgent specialist help is always required in this situation.

Aplastic crisis

This is potentially fatal. The erythrocyte count drops rapidly due to an infection with parvovirus.

The patient may present with:

- lethargy
- pallor
- severe anaemia
- blood film may reveal a raised INR and LFTs

Treatment is supportive and urgent specialist help is required.

ASSESSMENT

Prompt assessment is vital when dealing with sickle cell crisis. As always use a structured ABCDE approach.

Airway

- Assess and maintain airway.
- Utilise head tilt, chin lift if necessary.
- Use airway adjuncts if required.
- Consider urgent referral to anaesthetist for intubation if unable to protect airway.
- If the patient has signs of acute chest syndrome they are likely to need ventilation – call an anaesthetist now.

Breathing

- Assess oxygen saturations using pulse oximeter – aim to maintain saturations at 92–95%.
- Give high flow oxygen via non re-breath mask.
- Obtain arterial blood gases to assess oxygenation accurately and titrate oxygen therapy in accordance with results.
- Assess respiratory rate.
- Examine respiratory system.
- Request chest x-ray – look for signs of infiltrates.
- If infiltrates present on CXR treat for acute chest syndrome.
- Summon expert help.

Circulation

- Assess heart rate and rhythm.
- Record blood pressure.
- Record temperature.
- If temperature >38.5 °C this is an emergency.
- Obtain blood and urine culture.
- Obtain a throat swab.
- Commence a broad spectrum antibiotic until sensitivities known – the patient is at high risk from streptococcus pneumoniae infections.
- Obtain ECG.
- Gain IV access.
- Obtain venous blood for group and save, U&E, LFTs, INR, FBC and reticulocyte count.
- Give IV fluids – start with one litre normal saline over eight hours.
- Consider the need for blood transfusion – this is of particular importance if splenic sequestration or aplastic crisis is suspected.
- If you have not already done so, get expert help now.

Disability

- Assess conscious level using AVPU.
- Assess severity of pain.
- Ensure adequate analgesia is prescribed and administered:
  - ➤ if the pain is recurrent, determine the dose of opioid analgesia that the patient has previously required to relieve the pain
  - ➤ alternatively load the patient with IV morphine 5–10 mg
  - ➤ the dose should depend on:
    - the severity of the pain
    - the size of the patient
    - the patient's previous opioid experience.
- Do not give IM analgesia as it is poorly absorbed.
- The subcutaneous route can be used.
- Alternatively get expert help to administer patient controlled analgesia (PCA).
- Following administration of analgesia re-assess and titrate dose according to response.
- A non-steroidal anti-inflammatory may be a useful adjunct to opioids.

Exposure

- If you have not already done so, obtain a detailed history and undertake a full physical examination.

NEUTROPENIC SEPSIS

DEFINITION

Neutropenia occurs approximately 7–14 days after chemotherapy. As a result of this patients become more susceptible to infection. The risk of infection is greater the faster the rate of decline of the neutrophil count and the longer the duration of the neutropenia, especially if the neutropenia lasts for more than ten days.

Neurtopenic sepsis is an infection as a result of chemotherapy induced neutropenia. Life-threatening sepsis is more likely to occur when the neutrophil count is $<1 \times 109/l$.

SYMPTOMS AND SIGNS

Patients may present with the following:

- fever – temperature $>38\,°C$ for 1 hour or $>38.5\,°C$ on one occasion with neutrophil count $<1 \times 10^9/l$

- rigors
- signs of:
  - ➤ chest infection
  - ➤ urinary infection
  - ➤ Hickman line or central line infection
- sweating
- headache
- muscle pain
- diarrhoea
- vomiting

LIFE-THREATENING FEATURES

- hypoxia
- impaired renal function
- hypotension
- tachycardia
- respiratory rate >24 per minute
- systolic BP <90 mmHg

ASSESSMENT

Prompt assessment is vital when dealing with neutropenic sepsis. As always, use a structured ABCDE approach.

Airway

- Assess and maintain airway.
- Utilise head tilt, chin lift if necessary.
- Use airway adjuncts if required.
- Consider urgent referral to anaesthetist for intubation if unable to protect airway.

Breathing

- Assess oxygen saturations using pulse oximeter – aim to maintain saturations >92%.
- Give high flow oxygen via non re-breath mask if SaO2 <92%.
- Obtain arterial blood gases to assess oxygenation and lactate level.
- Assess respiratory rate.
- Examine respiratory system.
- Request chest x-ray – look for signs of infection.
- Summon expert help.

Circulation

- Assess heart rate and rhythm.
- Record blood pressure.
- Record temperature.
- Obtain blood and urine culture.
- Obtain a throat swab.
- Obtain swab from Hickman/central line.
- If the patient has diarrhoea, obtain stool sample for culture.
- Obtain ECG.
- Gain IV access if Hickman/central line unusable.
- Obtain venous blood for U&E, FBC, CRP, INR, LFTs.
- If patient dehydrated administer IV fluids – start with one litre normal saline over eight hours.
- Maintain strict fluid balance chart.
- If patient does not pass urine within three hours consider catheterisation.
- If you have not already done so, get expert help now.
- Commence IV antibiotics in accordance with local hospital policy. Antibiotic therapy may include:
  - ➢ piptazobactam 4.5 g IV every eight hours
  - ➢ gentamicin 5 mg/kg in 100 mls normal saline once daily.
- If penicillin allergy – ceftazidime 2 g IV every eight hours.

Disability

- Assess conscious level using AVPU.
- Monitor blood sugar.

Exposure

- If you have not already done so, obtain a detailed history and undertake a full physical examination.

BLOOD TRANSFUSION GUIDANCE

In 2002 the Department of Health issued a Health Service Circular entitled *Better Blood Transfusion*. This document paved the way for safer blood transfusion and reporting of adverse incidents as a result of blood transfusion.

Safe blood transfusion practice is supported by the Serious Hazards of Transfusion organisation (SHOT) based in Manchester. Both SHOT and the DOH have issued clear guidelines to enable safe transfusion practice.

As a nurse practitioner you will know when your patient requires a blood transfusion. This is likely to be in the emergency situation, such as the patient with a GI bleed rather that the planned situation. With the advent of independent nurse prescribing and the BNF opening up to these prescribers (see Chapter 13) one would assume that blood can be prescribed by an appropriately trained prescriber. This is not the case. Independent nurse prescribers cannot prescribe blood as it is not a drug. Many prescribers utilise supplementary prescribing to prescribe blood but in the emergency situation this is not helpful. It is therefore likely that a medical practitioner will prescribe the blood a patient requires. It may be sensible to assist practice by working with your local hospital Trust to develop a guideline which enables the prescribing of blood in the emergency situation.

What follows is a guide for the administration of blood and blood products.

THE PRESCRIPTION

- Ensure the need for the transfusion has been explained to the patient by the practitioner prescribing the blood.
- This conversation should be documented in the patient's medical record.
- Ideally the patient should be given written information regarding blood transfusions – check with local guidelines.
- Check the patient's:
  - ➢ surname
  - ➢ first name
  - ➢ hospital number.
- Ensure the type of blood product to be administered is prescribed.
- The quantity to be administered must be documented.
- The date and duration of infusion must be clearly documented.
- If furosemide is required the dose and route must be prescribed.

TAKING THE BLOOD SAMPLE

- Ensure the patient has an identification wrist band.
- Confirm the patient's details on their wrist band match those on the prescription.
- Ask the patient to state their first name and date of birth if possible.
- Obtain blood in the appropriate bottles in accordance with local policy.
- Always label the bottles at the patient's bedside.
- The request card should be signed by the practitioner who has requested the blood transfusion.

THE BEDSIDE CHECK

- Only registered medical practitioners and qualified nurses can administer blood and blood products.
- Two qualified staff must perform the bedside transfusion check.
- Ensure the patient's identification details match on:
  - ➢ the patient's wrist band

> the prescription chart
> the medical notes
> the information sheet accompanying the unit of blood to be transfused
> the compatibility label attached to the unit of blood.

- Ask the patient to state their first name and date of birth.
- Check the product pack number and blood group match those on the compatibility slip and label attached to the unit of blood.
- Check the expiry date on the unit of blood.
- Check the unit for signs of leakage.
- Check for signs of discoloration.
- Check for clot formation within the unit of blood.
- Transfusions of red cells must commence within 30 minutes of removal from the blood fridge.
- The transfusion must be completed within four hours.

ADMINISTERING THE TRANSFUSION

- Explain the procedure to the patient.
- Check the cannula.
- Flush the cannula with 0.9% sodium chloride.
- Record baseline temperature, pulse and blood pressure.
- Prime the giving set with 0.9% sodium chloride.
- Advise the patient that they should report any fever, itching, rashes, shortness of breath or general malaise to staff immediately.
- Commence the transfusion.
- Record the date and time of commencement of each unit transfused and stop time.
- Record temperature, pulse and blood pressure 15 minutes after commencement of unit and at the end of each unit.
- Maintain a fluid balance chart.
- Repeat the bedside check for each unit administered.
- Change the giving set after 12 hours or after three units of blood.

ADVERSE REACTIONS

Adverse reactions can be acute (at the time of infusion) or delayed (several days after infusion):

- Pyrexia is probably the most common reaction.
- If the temperature is $>1.5\,°C$ above normal administer paracetamol 1 g orally.
- If the transfusion is running at a rate faster than over four hours, slow it down to four hourly.
- Rerecord the temperature in one hour.
- If the temperature has fallen, continue the transfusion at the original rate.
- If the temperature has not fallen, stop the infusion and re-assess the patient.

Signs of a severe reaction are:

- pyrexia >1.5 °C above normal despite paracetamol
- hypotension
- tachycardia
- headache
- rash
- bleeding
- pain in abdomen
- pain in loin
- pain in chest
- shivering
- sweating
- dyspnoea
- patients may have a feeling of agitation and undue apprehension

In the event of a severe reaction:

- Stop the transfusion.
- Summon medical assistance.
- Treat septic shock as per Chapter 4.
- Obtain a post-transfusion group and save from a vein in the opposite arm to that of the transfusion.
- Return all blood products to the transfusion laboratory giving details of the reaction that has occurred.

BLOOD TRANSFUSION AND JEHOVAH'S WITNESSES

Jehovah's Witnesses believe that the Bible teaches them the following:

- Blood is sacred to God.
- Blood means life in God's eyes.
- Blood must not be eaten.
- Blood leaving the body of a human or animal must be disposed of.
- Christians must 'abstain' from blood and will receive good health if they do.
- Blood was reserved for only one special use, the atonement of sins.
- When a Christian abstains from blood they are expressing their faith that 'only the shed blood of Jesus can truly redeem them and save their life'.
- Even in an emergency it is not permissible to sustain a life with blood.
- The violation of the doctrine on blood is a serious offence and may lead to the person no longer being able to call themselves a Witness.

Certain medical procedures are prohibited according to Jehovah's Witness publications. Other procedures are left to the discretion of the individual to determine whether the planned procedure would be in violation of the doctrine on blood. The following are prohibited:

- Homologous whole blood transfusions, or transfusions using the stored blood of others.
- Autologous whole blood transfusions, or transfusions using one's own stored blood.
- Pre-operative collection of blood for re-infusion during or after surgery.

Jehovah's Witnesses are prohibited from receiving:

- red blood cells
- white blood cells
- platelets
- blood plasma

Products containing blood fractions are not prohibited but it is left to the individual to decide whether or not they believe receiving the product would be in violation of the doctrine on blood.

The following are not prohibited:

- haemoglobin
- interferons
- interlukins
- albumin
- globulins
- factor VIII
- erythropoietin (EPO)

The use of dialysis and cell savage is left to the individual to decide whether or not they wish to receive treatment.

Giving a Jehovah's Witness a blood transfusion against their wishes is assault and could result in prosecution. Even in an emergency if you know a patient to be a Jehovah's Witness and you administer a blood transfusion you could be held to account for assault. In the USA a physician was prosecuted for administering a blood transfusion to a patient in an emergency whom he knew to be a Jehovah's Witness. In the UK there have been no such cases to date.

Most Jehovah's Witnesses carry identification cards alerting health care staff to the fact and detailing what they are and are not willing to receive in an emergency. You must abide by these wishes.

When taking a history it is important to establish your patient's religion. If they state they are a Jehovah's Witness you must clarify what treatment they would be willing to receive. They have a right to change their decision at any stage of their treatment. Most hospitals now carry specific patient identification bands for Jehovah's Witnesses which state that they do not wish to receive blood and any other specific instructions. Ensure your patient is wearing one and that everyone caring for the patient knows what their express wishes are.

REFERENCES

Department of Health (2002) *Better Blood Transfusion*. Health Service Circular 2002/009. London: DoH.

Journal of Church and State (2005) Jehovah's Witnesses, blood transfusions and the tort of misrepresentation. *Journal of Church and State* 7(4) Autumn.

Kumar P and Clark M (2003) *Clinical Medicine*, 3rd edn. London: Saunders.

Longmore M, Wilkinson I and Török E (2001) *Oxford Handbook of Clinical Medicine*, 5th edn. Oxford: Oxford University Press.

National Heart Lung and Blood Institute (2002) *The Management of Sickle Cell Disease*, 4th edn. Bethesda, Maryland: NIH Publications.

Pizzo P (1999) Fever in immunocompromised patients. *New England Journal of Medicine* 341: 893–900.

Serious Hazards of Transfusion (2005) *Progress in Blood Safety in the UK*. Annual Report of 2004. Manchester: SHOT.

13   Advanced Practice

AN OVERVIEW OF ADVANCED PRACTICE

Nurse practitioner roles are inherent in practice in the United States of America. Over recent years these roles have developed across the United Kingdom. The Department of Health paved the way for role development with two key documents, *Making a Difference* (1999) and *The NHS Plan* (2000). The key message from both of these documents was the development of expert roles for senior nurses to enhance patient care.

One cannot discuss how nurse practitioners can enhance the quality of care for patients without first looking at what skills they should possess. A nurse practitioner should:

- be an expert in clinical practice
- possess research skills
- have a consultancy role
- be aware of social policy issues
- possess leadership skills
- have a role in education
- possess the ability to collaborate across and outside the organisation
- be aware of ethical and legal frameworks
- understand the professional agenda

This level of expertise is achieved through the practitioner's many years of experience in the clinical setting at a senior level. This expertise is augmented by education and training. This enables the practitioner to utilise their skills as a consultant and resource. An expert is by their very nature in possession of an in-depth knowledge of the broader picture of nursing. They are in possession of a greater understanding of the professional agenda and the role which they and others play. In clinical practice not only is a detailed knowledge of 'micro' health assessment issues necessary but it is also pertinent to have a greater understanding of the 'macro' issues and their effects on the population as a whole (Hamric 2005). Nurse practitioners have a leadership role, leading the way in developing others and empowering others to develop. Not only must the practitioner empower members of the multi-disciplinary team but they also have a responsibility to empower patients, families and carers to care for themselves and improve their quality of life.

One of the defining characteristics of the nurse practitioner is that they spend the majority of their time on 'hands on' clinical care. The essence of the role lies in the level of decision-making, not the level of technical skill required to carry out a task, however complex that task may be. It is the sound knowledge base that nurse practitioners possess from which independent diagnoses based on the clinical findings are made (Hamric 2005). Nurse practitioner roles blend aspects of medicine and nursing through a nursing perspective.

An important adage first mooted by George Castledine in 1995 is: 'Be certain that as you develop and expand your role it is to maximise nursing.' Therefore you become a 'maxi nurse and not a mini doctor'. If you remain true to this your role will develop appropriately and patient care will be enhanced.

In May 2006 following a period of consultation the Nursing and Midwifery Council issued a document which will pave the way for Advanced Nurse Practitioners (ANP) to be registered on a sub-part of the NMC register. As a result of this document a definition of advanced practice was issued, along with details of the knowledge and skills an ANP must possess.

The NMC defines advanced practitioners as:

> highly experienced, knowledgeable and educated members of the care team who are able to diagnose and treat your health care needs or refer you to an appropriate specialist if needed.

The NMC proposes an ANP is able:

- to carry out physical examinations
- to use their expert knowledge and clinical judgement to decide whether to refer patients for investigations and make diagnoses
- to decide on and carry out treatment, including the prescribing of medicines or refer patients to an appropriate specialist
- to use their extensive practice experience to plan and provide skilled and competent care to meet patients' health and social care needs, involving other members of the health care team as appropriate
- to ensure the provision of continuity of care including follow-up visits
- to assess and evaluate, with patients, the effectiveness of the treatment and care provided and make changes as needed
- to work independently, although often as part of a health care team which they will lead
- as a leader of the team, to make sure that each patient's treatment and care is based on best practice

Over the coming months and years we will see the nurse practitioner title protected with only those who have been through approved training programmes being able to call themselves practitioners. This will ensure a robust education system for budding practitioners and maintain public safety.

THE CHALLENGES OF ADVANCED PRACTICE

As roles develop, the nurse practitioner will face many challenges. These roles are becoming more common across hospital Trusts within the United Kingdom but they remain a relatively new concept. With all new roles there is an element of uncertainty. This uncertainty may be from practitioners as they break down traditional boundaries and develop and augment new skills. There is also likely to be a degree of uncertainty from colleagues. Nursing and medical colleagues may feel threatened by this new role. Nurses may be threatened because they see it as moving away from a traditional nursing model and medics because you are developing skills that traditionally have been in their domain.

It is the responsibility of the practitioner developing these new skills to be sensitive to colleagues' concerns but also to be prepared to stand up for and promote the positive influence the role can have on patient care. It will not necessarily be easy. You will be given a tough time by some colleagues but persevere and you will succeed. If you are facing a challenging time, utilise those colleagues who have been pivotal in developing the role. Visionary leadership will have got you this far and will get you through the challenging times.

Experience has shown that as long as you remain true to the nursing philosophy that has got you to this point in your career you will succeed and colleagues and patients will reap the benefits.

Role ambiguity can occur if there is uncertainty about the expectations of the practitioner (Chase et al. 1996). It is vital to ensure that both the practitioner and those who will manage the role are clear about roles and responsibilities. The nurse practitioner must have a clear vision of what is expected of them on a day to day basis if roles are to succeed. Meet regularly with your manager and address concerns or problems as they arise. It may be pertinent to develop a job plan. A job plan details where you should be and what you are expected to achieve every day. This gives structure to your working day for both the practitioner and colleagues and can act as a useful tool for personal reflection.

LEGAL PERSPECTIVE

In our personal lives we are bound to abide by the laws of the land. This responsibility extends naturally into professional life. The three key elements of the legal system are:

- criminal law (Statute) – an individual is innocent until proven guilty
- civil law (common law or case law)
  - ➢ negligence
  - ➢ trespass on property
  - ➢ trespass on the person
- European law – if Europe passes a law we have to incorporate it into our laws

As a practitioner you are both accountable and liable for your acts and omissions. This principle is a key element of the Code of Professional Conduct laid down by the Nursing and Midwifery Council (NMC) in 2004, but it is also laid down in law.

As a practitioner you are accountable to:

• your employer
• the NMC
• the public through criminal law
• patients through civil law – liability

Professional and legal accountability are in some ways heads and tails of the same coin, the positive and the negative. On the positive side patients see practitioners as knowledgeable, skilful and competent professionals. This is supported by professional accountability. Health professionals exercise their expertise and apply their skills, knowledge and competence to the benefit of the patient. The negative aspect of this accountability is the fact that practitioners can be sued for damages. However, on a positive note, previous case law supports professionals by stating who was or was not liable and why.

As practitioners nurses are professionally and legally accountable for their acts and omissions. When undertaking a new role it is vital that you are adequately trained and are in possession of the requisite knowledge and skills to undertake the role asked of you and are competent to do the job (Nursing and Midwifery Council 2004). Failure to act within your sphere of competence could result in a claim for negligence being made against you. Negligence was defined in a legal case (*Blyth v Birmingham Waterworks Co. 1986*) as being 'the omission to do something which a reasonable man would do, or do something which a prudent and reasonable man would not do'.

In 1957 the Bolam test set the standard against which a professional would be judged in a court of law. This judges a practitioner against 'the standard of the ordinary skilled man exercising or professing to have that skill'. In reality this means that an expert witness would be sought and the judge would seek to determine what is accepted nursing practice. As yet no case has been brought before the courts where a nurse has been working in an expanded role and a claim of negligence has been made. It is therefore difficult to hypothesise as to whom practitioners would be measured against, a doctor or another nurse, under these circumstances. The golden rule to follow as you develop your role as a practitioner is to ensure you are adequately trained to undertake what is expected of you. If you do not feel that you possess the knowledge and skills to undertake something, be it a clinical task or an aspect of assessment, do not do it until you feel that you do possess the requisite knowledge and skills.

ETHICAL PRINCIPLES

This section will attempt to give some guidance on ethical principles. There are many useful texts available to guide ethical decision-making, and the very nature of ethics means that no one text can be truly universal. The best advice to give if you have an interest in ethics is to read widely.

Ethics can be divided into three different catagories:

- professional ethics – the professional code of conduct
- societal ethics – the law
- medical ethics – autonomy, beneficence, non-maleficence, justice and veracity

What is important to remember is that modern health care gives rise to many value-laden issues for which nursing and medicine alone cannot provide an adequate answer.

Patients and their families may seek a solution to a problem that maximises the possibilities for a good outcome, or that fulfils their sense of duty to self and others, or that follows a rule or principle such as 'do unto others'. What is important to remember is that each ethical dilemma you come across is different and will need to be put into context for that particular patient, their expectations and their opinions and values. Each ethical question that arises can be examined under the spotlight of a number of different but not necessarily exclusive principles. They are:

- *Autonomy*: Patients have the right to choose actions that are consistent with their values, goals and life plan.
- *Beneficence*: Act in the best interests of the patient. We seek to provide a benefit for the patient in terms of the patient's goals.
- *Non-maleficence*: Do no harm.
- *Justice*: Treat persons fairly.
- *Veracity*: Be truthful and honest.

When it comes to ethical decision-making you may need to discuss the options and possible consequences of actions or inactions with colleagues. However, this is not always possible. Whenever you face a dilemma remember the following:

- What are the patient's wishes?
- Is what you are considering in the best interest of the patient and does it comply with the patient's wishes?
- What are the likely consequences of your actions or inactions?
- Is what you are considering equitable? Do not let external factors influence your decision.
- Does the patient know what all the options are and the possible benefits and possible side effects or risks of any treatment or investigation proposed?
- Do you have the knowledge and skills to undertake what is being asked of you?

If after working through this checklist you are still in doubt, seek advice from a colleague. It may be necessary at times to gain an expert legal opinion to ensure you are conforming to societal ethics.

Be reassured the ethical dilemma frequently challenges even the greatest minds. It is, after all, a dilemma. If after working through the dilemma you feel comfortable with the answer you reached, it is probably the right conclusion. If, however, you still feel uncomfortable with the decision it is probably best to discuss it with someone else. After all the discussions you may still feel uncomfortable. Sometimes the right decision for the patient is not what we would see as the correct professional decision; for example, when it comes to refusing treatment. Providing the patient has capacity and has made an informed decision, we sometimes have to stand back and remember that advocating for patients means that they make the decision that they feel is right for them and fits with their goals and life plan. After all, one of the main ethical principles is autonomy.

INFORMED CONSENT

The doctrine of informed consent has been developing in the United Kingdom since the 1980s. The legal rights of people in the UK result from various Acts of Parliament. In regards to healthcare patients have the following rights:

• the right to consent to treatment and research
• the right to refuse treatment and discharge oneself
• the right to receive relevant information before giving consent
• the right to receive the accepted standard of 'approved practice'
• the right to have confidential information kept confidential

Patients' autonomy must be respected at all times. This autonomy means they have the right to decide whether or not to undergo any investigation/intervention, even when a refusal may result in harm or in their own death. In order for a patient to exercise this right and to make informed decisions about their care they must be given sufficient information in a language that they can understand.

Practitioners working within the field of acute medicine are likely to be involved in gaining informed consent before procedures. If you are the practitioner undertaking the procedure, it is your responsibility to obtain consent prior to undertaking the procedure. If the procedure is being undertaken by someone else, you may obtain consent providing you have been trained to obtain consent for that particular procedure. If you have not been trained to undertake consent for a procedure you are not performing, you should not be attempting to obtain a patient's consent.

When obtaining consent it is the practitioner's responsibility to ensure they provide sufficient information to enable the patient to make a decision. Patients have a right to information about their condition and the treatment options available to them. The amount of information given may vary according to the patient's condition, the complexity of the treatment and the risk associated with the particular investigation or treatment that is proposed. When gaining consent the information given to a patient should include the following:

• details of the diagnosis and prognosis and the likely prognosis if the condition is left untreated

- uncertainties about the diagnosis including options for any further investigation prior to treatment
- options for treatment or management of the condition, including the option not to treat
- the purpose of a proposed investigation or treatment; this should include details of the procedure involved and information on what the patient might experience during and after a procedure
- for each option accompanying explanations of the likely benefits and the probabilities of success should be given; it is important to give the patient details of any serious or occurring risks associated with the investigation or procedure
- if a proposed treatment is experimental, advice must be given
- how and when the patient's condition and any side effects will be monitored or re-assessed
- the name of the doctor who will have overall responsibility for the treatment (usually the consultant)
- whether doctors or nurses in training will be involved
- a reminder that the patient can change their mind about a decision at any time
- a reminder that a patient has the right to seek a second opinion

You must not exceed the scope of authority given by the patient except in an emergency situation.

Answer any questions the patient may have honestly. Do not withhold information necessary for a patient to make an informed decision. Information can only be withheld if it is judged to cause the patient serious harm. This does not mean that the patient may become upset. If you are unsure, discuss this with a senior colleague and with the admitting consultant.

- No-one can make decisions on behalf of a competent adult.

In an emergency where consent cannot be obtained you may provide treatment to anyone who needs it, where it is necessary to save life.

ASSESSMENT OF CAPACITY

Practitioners should work on the principle that every adult has the capacity to make informed decisions about investigation and treatment unless it is shown that they cannot understand information that is presented to them in a clear and simple way. If you are unsure about a patient's capacity after you have presented them with the facts, it may be necessary to assess capacity formally. It is unlikely to be the remit of the nurse practitioner and local policies must be consulted as to the process for assessing capacity. The Code of Practice of the Mental Health Commission (1998) states that if a patient does not have capacity you may compulsorily treat them for a mental disorder only within the safeguards laid down in the Mental Health Act (1983) and any physical disorder arising from that mental disorder. It may be necessary to gain approval from the courts for any investigation or treatment outside of these parameters. The Mental Capacity Act (2005) gives guidance on the assessment of capacity and assessing the 'best interests' of a patient. Information on this Act can be found in the following section of this chapter.

Advanced directives or 'living wills' are becoming more common within the UK. If a patient is known to have issued an advanced directive you must respect any refusal of treatment. Failure to do so could result in legal action against the practitioner.

MENTAL CAPACITY ACT (2005)

After much controversy and media attention the Mental Capacity Act was published in 2005. This Act lays down the principles of assessment of capacity and the process that leads a person to be deemed as lacking the capacity to make decisions, be they decisions regarding the day to day functions of life or decisions pertaining to medical treatment. The Act states that a person lacks capacity in relation to a matter if at the material time they are unable to make a decision for themselves because of an impairment of, or a disturbance in, the functioning of the mind or brain. It does not matter whether the impairment or disturbance is permanent or temporary.

The following information on assessment of capacity is reproduced from the Mental Capacity Act (2005) and is subject to Crown Copyright.

The Act states that a person is unable to make a decision for themselves if they are unable to:

- understand the information relevant to the decision
- retain the information
- use or weigh that information as part of the process of making the decision
- communicate their decision whether by talking, using sign language or any other means

If a person is able to retain the information relevant to a decision for a short period only, they should be regarded as being able to make the decision.

The Act gives information on the determination of 'best interests'. In determining what is in a person's 'best interests', judgment must not be made merely on the basis of:

- the person's age or appearance
- a condition or aspect of behaviour which might lead others to make unjustified assumptions about what might be in their best interests

The person determining 'best interests' must consider all the relevant circumstances and in particular take the following steps:

- consider whether the person will at some time have capacity to make a decision
- ask, if it is likely that they will – when are they likely to have that capacity?

Where the determination of capacity relates to life-sustaining treatment, one must consider the following:

- the person's past and present wishes and feelings, if it is possible to ascertain these
- any relevant written statement made when they had capacity
- the views of the following, if this is practicable and appropriate:
  - anyone named by the person as someone who should be consulted
  - anyone engaged in caring for the person or interested in their welfare
  - anyone with lasting power of attorney granted by the person
  - any deputy appointed for the person by the court

Life-sustaining treatment is defined by the Act as treatment which in the view of a person providing healthcare for the person concerned is necessary to sustain life.

PRESCRIBING

Non-medical prescribing is a new concept in the UK. The Medicinal Products: Prescription by Nurses and Others Act 1992 paved the way for nurses to prescribe medicines. Since then non-medical prescribing has taken giant strides forward culminating in the amendments to medicine legislation (SI 2006/1015) which from May 2006 has allowed all registered independent prescribers to prescribe within their scope of practice from the British National Formulary (BNF) with the exception of most controlled drugs.

Non-medical prescribing has two components, independent and supplementary prescribing.

Independent prescribing entails the prescriber undertaking a patient assessment, diagnosing, making a balanced judgment as to the treatment options and prescribing the appropriate treatment.

Supplementary prescribing entails a doctor diagnosing the patient's condition and the doctor, the supplementary prescriber and the patient devising a management plan which enables the supplementary prescriber to titrate and adjust medication within clear parameters. This clinical management plan gives clear guidance as to when treatment can be amended, the dosage parameters and when to refer back to the independent prescriber. The supplementary prescriber cannot prescribe outside of this clinical management plan (CMP). Within an acute setting supplementary prescribing does not have a clear role as it relies on someone else diagnosing the patient and taking time to devise a plan. It is probably best suited to chronic disease management. However, it may have a place for the regular attender of the MAU. Patients that you know attend regularly despite all efforts to manage their condition in the community could potentially have a clinical management plan devised enabling the practitioner to assess the need for treatment and initiate certain therapies at an earlier stage in the assessment process. Many of these patients attend regularly due to chronic disease such as COPD. In these circumstances devising a CMP may be appropriate. Some examples of CMPs can be found in the Appendices.

The Nursing and Midwifery Council (2006) have issued standards for prescribing practice which all nurses who prescribe must adhere to. Some parts of this guidance are for NHS Trusts to follow; other parts apply to the individual prescriber.

The standards cover the issues of accountability, communication, consent and good prescribing practice. Many of these issues have been covered earlier in this chapter. The key principles to adhere to are:

- Remember that you are professionally accountable for your prescribing decisions and this accountability cannot be delegated.
- Before you prescribe you must have undertaken a full assessment of the patient.
- Only prescribe where there is a genuine need for treatment.
- Keep accurate, comprehensive records.
- Do not prescribe for yourself, family or friends unless there are exceptional circumstances.
- It is your responsibility to remain up to date to enable competent and safe prescribing.

Before nurses can independently prescribe the NMC has stated that the Trust for which they work must ensure that they are in possession of details of drugs that each individual is likely to prescribe. This is due to the fact that an individual prescriber is not going to prescribe freely from the whole BNF. Whilst it is acknowledged that an individual practitioner will only prescribe within their own level of knowledge, skill and competence in order to ensure protection under vicarious liability it is important that the NMC conditions are complied with. What form this compliance takes will vary from Trust to Trust. It is therefore vital that once registered as a prescriber you ascertain what local arrangements are in place for compliance with the NMC standards.

Deciding what you are likely to prescribe when working in the field of acute medicine is extremely difficult. By its very nature acute medicine covers a vast array of presenting complaints and co-morbidities for each patient. It may be easier to ascertain what you would not prescribe, i.e. what is outside of your scope of practice. Probably the easiest way to do this is to spend some time trawling through the BNF and coming up with a list of exclusions.

To help this process here are some suggestions as to drugs you may not want to prescribe:

- anabolic steroids
- prostoglandins and oxytocics
- intra-uterine devices
- intrathecal chemotherapy
- specialist drugs in neutropeonia
- total parenteral nutrition (TPN)
- drugs used in acute porphyria
- local corticosteroid injections
- antifungals for the eye

- local anaesthetics for the eye
- drugs for ocular diagnostic and peri-operative assessment and photodynamic treatment
- immunoglobulins in vaccination
- vaccinations for international travel
- intravenous anaesthetics
- inhalational anaesthetics
- non-opioid analgesics for use in anaesthesia
- opioid analgesics for use in anaesthesia
- muscle relaxants in anaesthesia
- anticholinesterases for use in anaesthesia
- drugs for the treatment of malignant hyperthermia in anaesthesia

Practitioners may decide that there are other groups of drugs which they would be unhappy to prescribe. This is a matter for individuals. A clause may be added to any documentation on what a practitioner will or will not prescribe, stating that any medication previously prescribed by a medical practitioner may be continued by the non-medical prescriber even if it is not in the pre-determined list of medications which they would normally prescribe. Finally, remember, just because your list says you can prescribe a certain drug it doesn't mean you are obliged to prescribe it if in your clinical judgment you do not believe it to be the correct treatment for a patient; after all, you are the only one who will be held to account if something goes wrong.

PATIENT GROUP DIRECTIONS

This is not concerned with prescribing but the supply and administration of medicines under specific circumstances. Circumstances under which a nurse may supply and administer a medication are clearly laid down in each individual PGD. Prior to use they are approved by senior doctors, pharmacists and nurses. The use of a PGD should not involve clinical judgement. A PGD applies to patients who have clearly defined similar medication requirements. Guidance on the writing of PGDs was given in HSC 2000/026.

PGDs are useful for the administration of drugs such as paracetamol and can be utilised by any nurse. Each PGD has very clear parameters for the supply and administration of a medicine and are very prescriptive. If a patient does not fulfil the criteria for use of the PGD then that PGD cannot be used. There is no room for clinical judgement.

While there is a definite role within acute medicine for the utilisation of PGDs, the nurse practitioner needs to be able to use their clinical judgement in order to function and therefore patient care would be enhanced by the undertaking of a prescribing course. However, on occasions a PGD may be useful; therefore examples of PGDs are included in the appendices.

CONCLUSION

Nurse practitioners are at the forefront of healthcare delivery. As traditional boundaries are eroded new and exciting opportunities are developing. It is up to nurses to seize these opportunities and drive change to ensure that patients receive high-quality care in an appropriate and timely manner, by a professional who is in possession of the requisite knowledge and skills.

BIBLIOGRAPHY

Due to the vast amount of literature pertaining to the areas covered in this chapter the following bibliography has been included.

Beauchamp T and Childress J (1994) *Principles of Biomedical Ethics*, 4th edn. Oxford: Oxford University Press.
Benner P (1984) *From Novice to Expert: Excellence and Power in Clinical Nursing*. Menlo Park: Addison-Wesley.
Bolam v. Friern HMC (1957) [2 All ER 188].
Casey and Smith (1997) Bringing nurses and doctors closer together. *British Medical Journal* 314: 617 (1 March).
Casteldine G (1995) Will the nurse practitioner be a mini doctor or maxi nurse? *British Journal of Nursing* 4(16): 938–9.
Casteldine G and McGee P (1998) *Advanced and Specialist Nursing Practice*. Oxford: Blackwell Science.
Department of Health (1992) *Medicinal Products: Prescription by Nurses and Others Act*. London: Stationery Office.
Department of Health (1999) *Making a Difference: Strengthening the Nursing, Midwifery and Health Visiting Contribution to Health and Healthcare*. London: Stationery Office.
Department of Health (2000) *The NHS Plan: A Plan for Investment, a Plan for Reform*. London: Stationery Office.
Dimond B (1996) *Mental Health Law for Nurses*. Oxford: Blackwell Science.
Dimond B (2001) *Legal Aspects in Nursing*, 3rd edn. London: Prentice Hall.
General Medical Council (1998) *Good Medical Practice*. London: GMC.
Gillon R (1994) *Principles of Health Care Ethics*. Chichester: Wiley & Son.
Green C (1999) When is a patient capable of consent? *Nursing Times* 95(6) (10 Feb).
Hamric A (2005) *Advanced Nursing Practice: An Integrative Approach*. London: WB Saunders.
Mayled A (1998) Medical admissions units: the role of the nurse practitioner. *Nursing Standard* 12(27): 44–7.
McGee D (1999) The legal framework for informed consent. *Professional Nurse* 14(10): 668–90.
Mental Health Commission (1998) *Code of Practice. Pursuant of S118 of the Mental Health Act 1983*.
NHSE ME (1991) *Junior Doctors: The New Deal*. London: Stationery Office.
Nursing and Midwifery Council (2004) *The NMC Code of Professional Conduct: Standards for Conduct, Performance and Ethics*. London: NMC.

Nursing and Midwifery Council (2006) *Standards for Prescribing Practice*. London: NMC.

Power K (1997) The legal and ethical implications of consent to nursing procedures. *British Journal of Nursing* 6(15): 885.

Rolfe G and Fulbrook P (1998) *Advanced Nursing Practice*. Oxford: Butterworth-Heinemann.

Scholefield H, Viney C and Evans J (1997) Expanding practice and obtaining consent. *Professional Nurse* 13(1): 12.

Sidani S and Irvine D (1999) A conceptual framework for evaluating the nurse practitioner role in acute care settings. *Journal of Advanced Nursing* 30(1): 58–66.

Woods L (1998) Identifying the practice characteristics of advanced practitioners in the acute care setting. *Intensive and Critical Care Nursing* 15: 308–17.

Appendix I   Examples of Clinical Management Plans

SEVERE ALCOHOL WITHDRAWAL (PATIENT <65 YEARS OF AGE NO LIVER DISEASE OR COPD)

Name of Patient: Unit Number: DOB:	Patient medication sensitivities/allergies:
Independent Prescriber:	Supplementary Prescriber:
Condition(s) to be treated Severe Alcohol withdrawal	Aim of treatment Minimise symptoms of withdrawal

Medicines that may be prescribed by SP: pabrinex, diazepam

Preparation	Indication	Dose schedule	Specific indications for referral back to the IP
Pabrinex	Moderate – severe alcohol withdrawal	1–2 pair of ampoules by IV infusion in 50–100 mls sodium chloride twice daily for 3 days. If symptoms persist continue with once daily until symptom free	If condition deteriorates or symptoms of alcohol withdrawal do not ease
Diazepam	Severe alcohol withdrawal	10 mg 6 hourly for 2 days then titrate down as per local guidelines. Plus 5–10 mg prn to a maximum of 40 mg in 24 hours	If symptoms persist

Guidelines or protocols supporting Clinical Management Plan:

Frequency of review and monitoring by Supplementary Prescriber and Independent Prescriber:

Process for reporting ADRs:
Patient to report any adverse effects to Supplementary Prescriber who will make initial decision to continue or stop medication depending on type of ADR.
In absence of Supplementary prescriber any ADR must be reported immediately to the on call doctor, Supplementary Prescriber or discuss with Independent Prescriber if unsure of the course of action to take.
If ADR results in stopping medication then Independent and Supplementary Prescribers must review management as soon as possible.
ADRs must be reported using the yellow card scheme by the Supplementary Prescriber.

Agreed by Independent Prescriber	Date	Agreed by Supplementary Prescriber	Date	Date agreed with patient/carer

ASTHMA

Name of Patient: Unit Number: DOB:	Patient medication sensitivities/allergies:
Independent Prescriber:	Supplementary Prescriber:
Condition(s) to be treated Asthma	Aim of treatment To minimise effects of an exacerbation of asthma and relieve breathlessness. Control and prevention of symptoms

Medicines that may be prescribed by SP: oxygen, prednisolone, ipratropium bromide nebuliser, beclomethasone inhaler, salmeterol inhaler, seretide inhaler

Preparation	Indication	Dose schedule	Specific indications for referral back to the IP
Oxygen 24–100%	Hypoxia (oxygen saturations <92%)	Titrated to maintain saturations of at least 92%	If asthma control deteriorates or does not respond to treatment
Ipratropium bromide nebuliser	Exacerbation of asthma	250–500 micrograms 4 times daily	
Beclomethasone inhaler	Exacerbation prevention	100–400 micrograms twice daily	
Salmeterol	Long acting bronchodilation	25–100 micrograms twice daily	
Seretide inhaler	To minimise number of inhalers and improve asthma control prior to discharge	50–500 micrograms twice daily	

Guidelines or protocols supporting Clinical Management Plan: BTS/SIGN (2003) British Guideline on the management of Asthma. *Thorax* Vol. 38 Suppl. 1

Frequency of review and monitoring by Supplementary Prescriber and Independent Prescriber:

Process for reporting ADRs:
Patient to report any adverse effects to Supplementary Prescriber who will make initial decision to continue or stop medication depending on type of ADR.
In absence of Supplementary Prescriber any ADR must be reported immediately to the on call doctor. Supplementary Prescriber to discuss with Independent Prescriber if unsure of the course of action to take.
If ADR results in stopping medication then Independent and Supplementary Prescribers must review management as soon as possible.
ADRs must be reported using the yellow card scheme by the Supplementary Prescriber.

Agreed by Independent Prescriber	Date	Agreed by Supplementary Prescriber	Date	Date agreed with patient/carer

COPD

Name of Patient: Unit Number: DOB:	Patient medication sensitivities/allergies:
Independent Prescriber:	**Supplementary Prescriber:**
Condition(s) to be treated Exacerbation of COPD	**Aim of treatment** To minimise effects of an exacerbation of COPD and ease acute breathlessness. Symptom control

Medicines that may be prescribed by SP: oxygen, prednisolone, salbutamol, atrovent, beclomethasone, salmeterol, seretide

Preparation	Indication	Dose schedule	Specific indications for referral back to the IP
Oxygen	Hypoxia	24–40%. Titrate according to ABGs and monitor for CO_2 retention	If no response to treatment or condition deteriorates
Prednisolone	Exacerbation of COPD	30 mg once daily or increase usual dose by 30 mg	
Salbutamol nebuliser	Exacerbation of COPD	2.5–5 mg qds and prn	
Salbutamol inhaler	Symptom control	2 puffs prn	
Ipratropium bromide nebuliser	Symptom control	250–500 micrograms qds	
Ipratropium bromide inhaler	Symptom control	20–40 micrograms qds	
Beclomethasone	Prevention of exacerbations	100–400 micrograms qds	
Salmeterol inhaler	Prevention of exacerbations	25–100 micrograms twice daily	
Seretide inhaler	Prevention of exacerbations	50–500 micrograms twice daily	

Guidelines or protocols supporting Clinical Management Plan:
NICE (2004) Chronic Obstructive Pulmonary Disease. Management of chronic obstructive pulmonary disease in primary and secondary care. Clinical Guideline 12

Frequency of review and monitoring by Supplementary Prescriber and Independent Prescriber:

Process for reporting ADRs:
Patient to report any adverse effects to Supplementary Prescriber who will make initial decision to continue or stop medication depending on type of ADR.
In absence of Supplementary Prescriber any ADR must be reported immediately to the on call doctor.
Supplementary Prescriber to discuss with Independent Prescriber if unsure of the course of action to take.
If ADR results in stopping medication then Independent and Supplementary Prescribers must review management as soon as possible.
ADRs must be reported using the yellow card scheme by the Supplementary Prescriber.

Agreed by Independent Prescriber	Date	Agreed by Supplementary Prescriber	Date	Date agreed with patient/carer

PARACETAMOL OVERDOSE

Name of Patient: Unit Number: DOB:	Patient medication sensitivities/allergies:
Independent Prescriber:	Supplementary Prescriber:
Condition(s) to be treated Paracetamol overdose	Aim of treatment Minimise effects of overdose

Medicines that may be prescribed by SP: acetylcysteine, chlorphemiramine, hydrocortisone

Preparation	Indication	Dose schedule	Specific indications for referral back to the IP
Acetylcysteine	If paracetamol levels slightly below or above the treatment line as per Clinical Guidelines	150 mg per kg in 200 mls of 5% glucose over 15 minutes; then 50 mg per kg in 500 mls 5% glucose over 4 hours; then 100 mg per kg in 1 litre of 5% glucose over 16 hours. Repeat investigations. If has or remains at risk of fulminant hepatic failure give further 50 mg per kg in 500 mls of 5% glucose over 8 hours	If shows signs of fulminant hepatic failure and/or requires a further bag of acetylcysteine after 16 hour bag
Chlorpheniramine	If shows signs of pseudo-allergic reaction to acetylcysteine	10 mg IV over 1 minute	If signs of pseudo-allergic reaction do not subside
Hydrocortisone	If shows signs of pseudo-allergic reaction to acetylcysteine	100 mg IV up to four times daily	If signs of pseudo-allergic reaction do not subside

Guidelines or protocols supporting Clinical Management Plan:
Toxbase accessed via www.spib.axl.co.uk

Frequency of review and monitoring by Supplementary Prescriber and Independent Prescriber:

Process for reporting ADRs:
Patient to report any adverse effects to Supplementary Prescriber who will make initial decision to continue or stop medication depending on type of ADR.
In absence of Supplementary Prescriber any ADR must be reported immediately to the on call doctor.
Supplementary Prescriber to discuss with Independent Prescriber if unsure of the course of action to take.
If ADR results in stopping medication then Independent and Supplementary Prescribers must review management as soon as possible.
ADRs must be reported using the yellow card scheme by the Supplementary Prescriber.

Agreed by Independent Prescriber	Date	Agreed by Supplementary Prescriber	Date	Date agreed with patient/carer

PULMONARY EMBOLISM

Name of Patient: Unit Number: DOB:	Patient medication sensitivities/allergies:
Independent Prescriber:	**Supplementary Prescriber:**
Condition(s) to be treated Pulmonary Embolism	**Aim of treatment** Ensure prophylaxis until PE confirmed. Once confirmed, to treat PE

Medicines that may be prescribed by SP: dalteparin, warfarin, oxygen, indomethacin

Preparation	Indication	Dose schedule	Specific indications for referral back to the IP
Oxygen	Shortness of breath and hypoxia due to suspected PE	24–100% titrated to maintain oxygen saturation >95%	If hypoxia persists
Dalteparin	Suspected PE and maintenance of anticoagulation prior to INR becoming therapeutic	7,500–18,000 units once daily	Patient demonstrates bleeding tendencies
Warfarin	Confirmed PE	Titrated according to INR	INR not stabilising
Indomethacin	Chest pain prior to PE being confirmed. Once confirmed and warfarin commenced this must be stopped	25–50 mg tds	Pain is uncontrolled

Guidelines or protocols supporting Clinical Management Plan:
British Thoracic Society (2003) Guidelines for the management of suspected acute pulmonary embolism. *Thorax* 58: 470–484

Frequency of review and monitoring by Supplementary Prescriber and Independent Prescriber:

Process for reporting ADRs:
Patient to report any adverse effects to Supplementary Prescriber who will make initial decision to continue or stop medication depending on type of ADR.
In absence of Supplementary Prescriber any ADR must be reported immediately to the on call doctor.
Supplementary Prescriber to discuss with Independent Prescriber if unsure of the course of action to take.
If ADR results in stopping medication then Independent and Supplementary Prescribers must review management as soon as possible.
ADRs must be reported using the yellow card scheme by the Supplementary Prescriber.

Agreed by Independent Prescriber	Date	Agreed by Supplementary Prescriber	Date	Date agreed with patient/carer

SEVERE ANAEMIA

Name of Patient:	Patient medication sensitivities/allergies:
Unit Number: DOB:	

Independent Prescriber:	Supplementary Prescriber:

Condition(s) to be treated	Aim of treatment
Severe Anaemia	Symptomatic treatment of anaemia

Medicines that may be prescribed by SP: blood transfusion, furosemide, hydroxocobalamin, oxygen

Preparation	Indication	Dose schedule	Specific indications for referral back to the IP
Oxygen	Shortness of breath	24–60% titrated to maintain arterial oxygen saturation >92%	If patient remains symptomatic despite treatment
Blood transfusion	Symptomatic anaemia	2–4 units each given over 4 hours (rarely >2–3 units in 24 hours)	
Furosemide	Prevention of fluid overload with blood transfusion	20–40 mg with alternate units of blood	If develops signs of overload despite furosemide
Hydroxocobalamin	Macrocytic anaemia due to B12 deficiency	1 mg IM on alternate days for 6 doses	

Guidelines or protocols supporting Clinical Management Plan:
Department of Health (2002) Better Blood Transfusion. Health Service Circular 2002/009. DOH: London

Frequency of review and monitoring by Supplementary Prescriber and Independent Prescriber:

Process for reporting ADRs:
Patient to report any adverse effects to Supplementary Prescriber who will make initial decision to continue or stop medication depending on type of ADR.
In absence of Supplementary Prescriber any ADR must be reported immediately to the on call doctor.
Supplementary Prescriber to discuss with Independent Prescriber if unsure of the course of action to take.
If ADR results in stopping medication then Independent and Supplementary Prescribers must review management as soon as possible.
ADRs must be reported using the yellow card scheme by the Supplementary Prescriber.

Agreed by Independent Prescriber	Date	Agreed by Supplementary Prescriber	Date	Date agreed with patient/carer

Appendix II　Examples of Patient Group Directions

FUROSEMIDE PGD

Medicine and PGD number　　Intravenous furosemide 40 mg (4 mls)

Dose, route and duration
40 mg in 4 mls via intravenous injection at a rate of 4 mg / min as a once only dose

Legal Status Prescription only medicine

Reference Number

Date PGD comes into force

Date PGD expires

Clinical condition/situation for which the PGD applies
Patients with clinical features of left ventricular failure

Criteria for confirmation of the clinical condition/situation
Assessment by an appropriately trained nurse practitioner

Further advice/referral in any of the following situations
Liver failure LFTs >25% normal range
Deranged urea and electrolyte results – creatinine >150

Exclusion criteria
Precomatose states associated with cirrhosis of the liver
Renal failure with anaemia
Previous adverse reactions to furosemide
Pregnancy and breast feeding
Hypotension – diastolic BP <50 mm Hg
Porphyria

Actions to be followed for patients excluded from the PGD
Discuss with medical practitioner, ensure all alternative treatments are explored
Details of action to be taken for patients who do not wish to receive or do not adhere to care under the PGD
• Discuss all treatment options
• Ensure informed decision
• Record in client records
• Inform medical practitioner

Potential adverse reactions
• Hypotension
• Hypomagnesaemia
• Nausea
• Gastro-intestinal disturbances
• Gout
• Hypoglycaemia
• Tinnitus
• Rashes
• Shock

The following can occur but are unlikely after a single dose:

• Hyponatraemia
• Hypokalaemia
• Hypomagnesaemia
• Increased calcium secretion
• Bone marrow depression

Procedure to follow when dealing with an adverse reaction
• Stop medication
• Seek medical review as appropriate

Patient monitoring parameters/special instructions
• Monitor the effectiveness of the drug – i.e. do the patient's symptoms improve?
• If not already catheterised then do so and monitor hourly urine output
• Monitor blood pressure
• Record oxygen saturations
• If the patient's symptoms do not respond to this treatment they must be referred to a medical practitioner immediately

Patient information/advice to be given (e.g. authorised patient information leaflets/follow up treatments)
• Inform the patient they have been given a diuretic

REFERENCES

ABPI (2002) *Compendium of Data Sheets and Summaries of Product Characteristics*. Datapharm Publications Ltd.

British National Formulary (2006) 51st edn.

GTN PGD

Medicine and PGD number
Glyceryl trinitrate (GTN) 500 microgram tablet

Intended Client Group Adult/Child or both Adults

Dose, route and duration
- Glyceryl trinitrate (GTN) 500 mcg tablet
- Placed under the tongue (sub-lingual) and allowed to dissolve (DO NOT SWALLOW)
- A further tablet may be administered after 5 minutes
- A maximum of 3 doses can be administered under this PGD

GTN is readily absorbed from the oral mucosa and rapidly metabolised. The effects should be seen within 2–3 minutes

---

Legal Status
Pharmacy only medicine

Reference Number

Date PGD comes into force

Date PGD expires

Route and recording of the medication
- Record medication on patient's prescription chart as per Trust policy
- Document action in medical and nursing records

Type of health professional administering this medication
- Registered Nurse deemed competent in the administration of this medicine

---

Clinical condition/situation for which the PGD applies
- Acute chest pain of cardiac origin

Criteria for confirmation of the clinical condition/situation
- Patient has chest pain that is thought to be cardiac in origin
- Patient may have a history of ischaemic heart disease/angina or previous myocardial infarction
- An ECG may show signs of ischaemia or infarction

Refer to medical staff for further advice/referral in any of the following situations
- Pregnancy/lactation
- Urgent referral to medical staff must be made if the nurse suspects the patient may be having a myocardial infarction

Criteria for exclusion
- Known hypersensitivity to nitrates
- Head trauma
- Cerebral haemorrhage
- Closed-angle glaucoma
- Patients taking sildenafil – concurrent use contra-indicated due to additive hypotensive effects

Actions to be followed for patients excluded from the PGD
- Refer for urgent medical review

Actions to be taken for patients who decline treatment or do not adhere to care under the PGD
- Refer for urgent medical review

Potential adverse reactions
- Throbbing headache
- Facial flushing
- Dizziness
- Feeling of weakness
- Postural hypotension
- Tachycardia

Procedure to follow when dealing with an adverse reaction
- Inform medical practitioner immediately
- Complete Trust adverse incident report
- If adverse reaction is serious, complete Committee on Safety of Medicines Yellow Card

Patient monitoring parameters/special instructions
- The nurse will establish that pain is likely cardiac in origin
  - ➢ pain may be described as crushing, a tight band or a pressure on the chest and may radiate to the jaw or left arm
  - ➢ pain may be associated with sweating, nausea and vomiting
- An ECG must be obtained
- Record patient's heart rate and blood pressure
- Administer high flow oxygen (100%) via re-breathe mask unless the patient is known to retain CO_2, in which case give 2 litres of oxygen via mask (24%)

Following administration:
- Monitor effectiveness of treatment
- If pain persists after 5 minutes give a further dose to a maximum of 3 doses
- Record patients blood pressure and heart rate
- Consider administration of aspirin using aspirin PGD
- Refer to medical practitioner if pain unresolved

Patient information/advice to be given (e.g. authorised patient information)
- Explain the treatment and the course of action being taken

REFERENCES

ABPI (2002) *Compendium Data Sheets and Summaries of Product Characteristics*. DataPharm Publications.
British National Formulary (2006) 51st edn.

NALOXONE PGD

Medicine and PGD number Naloxone hydrochloride 400 mcg in 1 ml

Dose, route and duration 800 mcg via intravenous or intramuscular route every 2–3 minutes to a maximum of 10 mg

Legal Status Prescription only medicine

Reference Number

Date PGD comes into force

Date PGD expires

Clinical condition/situation for which the PGD applies For the complete or partial reversal of opioid induced respiratory depression

Criteria for confirmation of the clinical condition/situation • Opioids have recently been administered and/or patient is believed to have self administered opioids • One or more of the following are present: • Respiratory rate <6 per minute with poor tidal volume • Patient is unresponsive with Glasgow Coma Score of <8 out of 15 • Respiratory arrest • Pin point pupils

Further advice/referral in any of the following situations If patient is known to be dependent on opioids Contact medical team immediately if patient is not responding to naloxone treatment

Exclusion criteria Cardiovascular disease Physical dependence on opioids Known hypersensitivity to naloxone Known renal and/or hepatic impairment

Actions to be followed for patients excluded from the PGD
Immediate referral to medical staff
Details of action to be taken for patients who do not wish to receive or do not adhere to care under the PGD
The patient is unresponsive and therefore unable to refuse treatment in this emergency situation

Potential adverse reactions
• Nausea and vomiting
• Tachycardia
• Ventricular fibrillation
• Hyperventilation
• Hypertension
• Tremulousness
• Cardiac arrest

Procedure to follow when dealing with an adverse reaction
• Inform medical staff immediately
• Complete adverse incident form
• Document in medical and nursing notes

Patient monitoring parameters/special instructions
Doses will be administered until:
Patient's respiratory rate is above 12 per minute and oxygen saturation >90%

The following may also be seen following administration:
Patient's Glasgow Coma Score is >13 out of 15
Pupil size is no longer pin point

Patients having naloxone must be monitored via a defibrillator, pulse oximeter and blood pressure monitoring

The duration of some opioids may exceed that of naloxone and therefore the patient must be continuously monitored

If the administration of naloxone does not result in an improvement in the patient's condition they must be referred to the medical practitioner immediately

Patient information/advice to be given (e.g. authorised patient information leaflets/follow up treatments)
Inform them that they have had the effects of opioids reversed

REFERENCES

ABPI (2002) *Compendium of Data Sheets and Summaries of Product Characteristics*. Data-
    Pharm Publications.
British National Formulary (2006) 51st edn.

PARACETAMOL PGD

Medicine and PGD number	Paracetamol suspension 120 mg/5 ml Paracetamol suspension 250 mg/5 ml Paracetamol tablets 500 mg

Dose, route and duration
- Paracetamol suspension 250 mg/5 ml or paracetamol tablets 500 mg
1–2 tablets 6 hourly maximum 4 grams in 24 hours

Legal Status Pharmacy only medicine

Reference Number

Date PGD comes into force

Date PGD expires

Clinical condition/situation for which the PGD applies
Mild to moderate pain or prior to painful procedures

Criteria for confirmation of the clinical condition/situation
Assessment of pain score as per pain management protocol

Further advice/referral in any of the following situations
- History of severe liver or renal disease
- Patient taking cholestyramine (it inhibits the absorption of paracetamol)
- Patient displaying depressive/suicidal tendencies

Exclusion criteria
- Known hypersensitivity
- Paracetamol–containing product has been taken within the last 4–6 hours

Actions to be followed for patients excluded from the PGD
Discuss with medical practitioner, ensure all alternative treatment explored

Details of action to be taken for patients who do not wish to receive or do not adhere to care under the PGD
- Discuss all treatment options
- Ensure informed decision
- Record in client's records, inform medical practitioner

Potential adverse reactions
- Nausea, rashes
- Rarely acute pancreatitis after prolonged use

Procedure to follow when dealing with an adverse reaction
- Stop medication
- Follow anaphylaxis protocol as appropriate
- Seek medical review

Patient monitoring parameters/special instructions
- Review pain assessment to ensure adequate response to medication, particularly if prior to painful procedure. Seek medical review if not responsive
- Ensure the drug, dose and route are recorded in the client's notes

Patient information/advice to be given (e.g. authorised patient information leaflets/follow up treatments)
- Advise on maximum dosage and frequency of administration as stated above

REFERENCES

ABPI (2003) *Compendium of Data Sheets and Summaries of Product Characteristics*. Datapharm Publications.
British National Formulary (2006) 51st edn.

Glossary

A&E	accident and emergency
ABCDE	airway, breathing, circulation, disability, exposure
ACE	angiotensin converting enzyme
ACS	acute coronary syndrome
ACTH	adrenocorticotrophic hormone
AF	atrial fibrillation
ALS	advanced life support
ALT	alanine aminotransferase
ANP	advanced nurse practitioner
APTT	activated partial thrombin time
ARDS	acute respiratory distress syndrome
ARF	acute renal failure
AV	atrio ventricular
AVPU	alert, voice, pain, unresponsive
bd	bis die (twice a day)
BLS	basic life support
BMA	British Medical Association
BMI	body mass index
BNF	British National Formulary
BP	blood pressure
bpm	beats per minute
BSR	British Society of Rheumatology
BTS	British Thoracic Society
Ca_2	calcium
CMP	clinical management plan
CO_2	carbon dioxide
COPD	chronic obstructive pulmonary disease
CPR	cardiopulmonary resuscitation
CRP	C-reactive protein
CRT	capillary refill time
CSF	cerebrospinal fluid
CT	computerised tomography
CTPA	computerised tomography pulmonary angiogram
CURB 65	confusion, urea, respiratory rate, blood pressure, age $\geq$ 65
CVA	cerebrovascular accident
CVP	central venous pressure
CXR	chest x-ray

DIC	disseminated intravascular coagulation
DIGAMI	diabetes and insulin-glucose infusion in acute myocardial infarction
DKA	diabetic ketoacidosis
DNAR	do not attempt resuscitation
DOH	Department of Health
DVLA	Driver and Vehicle Licensing Authority
DVT	deep vein thrombosis
ECG	electrocardiogram
ECMO	extra corporeal membrane oxygenation
EPO	erythropoietin
ESR	erythrocyte sedementation rate
FBC	full blood count
FEV1	forced expiratory volume in 1 second
FOB	faecal occult blood
g	grams
g/dl	grams per decilitre
GCS	Glasgow coma scale
GI	gastro intestinal
GMC	General Medical Council
GP	general practitioner
GTN	glyceryl trinitrate
GU	genitourinary
Hb	haemoglobin
HbA	haemoglobin A
Hb Beta Thal	sickle beta thalassaemia
HbSS	sickle cell anaemia
HCO_3	bicarbonate
HIV	human immunodeficiency virus
HR	heart rate
HSC	health service circular
ICP	intracranial pressure
ICU/ITU	intensive care/therapy unit
IE	infective endocarditis
IgE	immunoglobulin E
IM	intramuscular
INR	international normalised ratio
IV	intravenous
JVP	jugular venous pressure
K	potassium
KCl	potassium chloride
kg	kilograms
kPa	kilopascal
LACS	lacunar syndrome

GLOSSARY

257

LBBB	left bundle branch block
LDH	lactate dehydrogenase
LFTs	liver function tests
LMA	laryngeal mask airway
LMWH	low molecular weight heparin
LOC	loss of consciousness
LP	lumbar puncture
LSD	lysergide
LV	left ventricle
MAU	medical assessment unit
mcg	micrograms
MCV	mean cell volume
mg	milligrams
MI	myocardial infarction
ml	millilitres
mmHg	millimetres of mercury
mmols	millimols
MONA	morphine, oxygen, nitrate, aspirin
MRI	magnetic resonance imaging
MSU	mid-stream urine
Na	sodium
NG	naso-gastric
NHS	National Health Service
NICE	National Institute for Clinical Excellence
NIV	non-invasive ventilation
NMC	Nursing and Midwifery Council
NSF	National Service Framework
NSTEMI	non ST elevation myocardial infarction
O_2	oxygen
od	omni die (once daily)
P	pulse
PA	posterior anterior
$PaCO_2$	partial pressure of carbon dioxide in arterial blood
PACS	partial anterior circulation syndrome
PaO_2	partial pressure of oxygen in arterial blood
PCA	patient controlled analgesia
PCR	polymerase chain reaction
PE	pulmonary embolism
PEA	pulseless electrical activity
PEFR	peak expiratory flow rate
PGD	Patient Group Direction
PND	paroxysmal nocturnal dyspnoea
POCS	posterior circulation syndrome
PPI	proton pump inhibitor

PR	per rectum
qds	quarter die sumendus (to be taken four times a day)
RCN	Royal College of Nurses
RCP	Royal College of Physicians
RR	respiratory rate
RSI	rapid sequence induction
SAH	subarachnoid haemorrhage
SaO_2	saturated oxygen
SERM	selective estregen receptor modulator therapy
SHOT	serious hazards of transfusion
SIADH	syndrome of inappropriate antidiuretic hormone secretion
SOAPIE	subjective, objective, assess, plan, implement, evaluate
SOCRATES	site, onset, character, radiation, associated features, timing, exacerbating/relieving factors, severity
STEMI	ST elevation myocardial infarction
SVT	supra ventricular tachycardia
TACS	total anterior circulation syndrome
TB	tuberculosis
TFT	Thyroid Function Tests
TIA	transient iscahemic attack
TPR	temperature, pulse, respiration
U&E	urea and electrolytes
UC	ulcerative colitis
UK	United Kingdom
USA	United States of America
UTI	urinary tract infection
VF	ventricular fibrillation
VQ	ventilation perfusion
VT	ventricular tachycardia
WBC	white blood (cell) count

Index